.

BIOMEDICAL & NANOMEDICAL TECHNOLOGIES
CONCISE MONOGRAPH SERIES

Basic Principles and Potential Applications of Holographic Microwave Imaging

Lulu Wang

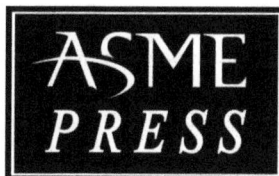

ASME PRESS

Library of Congress Cataloging-in-Publication Data

Names: Wang, Lulu, author.
Title: Basic principles and potential applications of holographic microwave imaging / Lulu Wang.
Description: New York : ASME Press, [2016] | Includes bibliographical references.
Identifiers: LCCN 2016025394 | ISBN 9780791860434
Subjects: LCSH: Microwave imaging in medicine. | Breast--Cancer--Diagnosis.
Classification: LCC RC78.7.M53 W36 2016 | DDC 616.07/54--dc23 LC record available at https://lccn.loc.gov/2016025394

Series Editors' Preface

Biomedical and Nanomedical Technologies (B&NT)
This **concise** monograph series focuses on the implementation of various engineering principles in the conception, design, development, analysis and operation of biomedical, biotechnological and nanotechnology systems and applications. The primary objective of the series is to compile the latest research topics in biomedical and nanomedical technologies, specifically devices and materials.

Each volume comprises a collection of invited manuscripts, written in an accessible manner and of a concise and manageable length. These timely collections will provide an invaluable resource for initial enquiries about technologies, encapsulating the latest developments and applications with reference sources for further detailed information. The content and format have been specifically designed to stimulate further advances and applications of these technologies by reaching out to the non-specialist across a broad audience.

Contributions to *Biomedical and Nanomedical Technologies* will inspire interest in further research and development using these technologies and encourage other potential applications. This will foster the advancement of biomedical and nanomedical applications, ultimately improving healthcare delivery.

Editor:
Ahmed Al-Jumaily, PhD, Professor of Biomechanical Engineering & Director of the Institute of Biomedical Technologies, Auckland University of Technology.

Associate Editors:
Christopher H.M. Jenkins, PhD, PE, Professor and Head, Mechanical & Industrial Engineering Department, Montana State University.

Said Jahanmir, PhD, President & CEO, MiTiHeart Corporation.

Shanzhong (Shawn) Duan, PhD, Professor, Mechanical Engineering, South Dakota State University.

Conrad M. Zapanta, PhD, Associate Department Head of Biomedical Engineering, Teaching Professor of Biomedical Engineering, Carnegie Mellon University.

William J. Weiss, PhD, Professor of Surgery and Bioengineering, College of Medicine, The Pennsylvania State University.

Siddiq M. Qidwai, PhD, Mechanical Engineer, U.S. Naval Research Laboratory.

Contents

Abstract

This monograph offers comprehensive descriptions of the most important principles so far proposed for far-field holographic microwave imaging—including reconstruction procedures and imaging systems and apparatus—enabling the reader to use microwaves for diagnostic purposes in a wide range of applications. This hands-on resource features:

+ A review of the existing medical imaging methods-including theory, apparatus and challenges, introducing some new medical imaging techniques.
+ A review of the existing microwave imaging techniques-including theory, apparatus, medical applications and challenges, written from an engineering perspective and with notations.
+ Currently proposed holographic microwave imaging technique-including reconstruction procedures and imaging systems and apparatus-enabling the reader to use microwaves for diagnostic purposes in a wide range of applications.
+ A discussion of practical applications with detailed descriptions and discussions of several specific examples (e.g., imaging dielectric object, small inclusion detection, and medical applications).
+ A conclusion of the proposed holographic microwave imaging technique and discussions of future research directions.

List of Symbols and Abbreviations

Symbols

k_0	Free-space propagation
k_b	Wavenumber of host medium
$\varepsilon(s)$	Complex relative permittivity distribution inside the dielectric object
ε_b	Relative permittivity of the host medium
ε_∞	Infinite frequency dielectric constant
ε_s	Static dielectric constant
ε_0	Permittivity of free-space
ε^*	The complex dielectric constant
τ	Characteristic relaxation time of the medium
σ	Conductivity of the tissue
ω	Angle frequency
E_{inc}	Incident electric field
E_{scat}	Backscattered electric field
$E_{tot}(s)$	Total electric field at a point inside the object with position vector, **s**
E_0	Wave amplitude of TE_{10} mode at within waveguide aperture
λ_b	Wavelength in the host medium
$\hat{R}$	Unit vector parallel to the vector R
R	Position vector from a point in the object to the selected receiver
R	Distance from a point in the object to the receiver
R_0	Distance from a point in the object to the transmitter
A	Narrow aperture dimension of antenna aperture
B	Broad aperture dimension of antenna aperture
$b(\theta,\varnothing)$	Radiation pattern function
$P(\theta,\varnothing)$	Polarization vector
$H_0^2(k_b R)$	Zero-order Hankel function of the second type with argument $k_b R$
$H_1^2(k_b R)$	First-order Hankel function of the second type with argument $k_b R$
dA	Differential area element
$[I]$	Identity matrix
$[M]$	Square matrix
D	Baseline vector
ΔS	Small area element

Abbreviations

2D	Two Dimensional
3D	Three Dimensional
BLOD	Blood Oxygen Level Dependent
CSF	Cerebral Spin Fluid
CT	Computed Tomography
EM	Electromagnetic
HMI	Holographic Microwave Imaging
IFFT	Inverse Fast Fourier Transform
IHM	Indirect Holography Microwave
MIST	Microwave Imaging Via Space Time
MoM	Method of Moment
MRI	Magnetic Resonance Imaging
ORWA	Open-ended Rectangular Waveguide Antenna
PET	Positron Emission Tomography
SNR	Signal Noise Ratio
TSAR	Tissue Sensing Adaptive Radar
US	Ultrasound
UWB	Ultra-Wideband
VNA	Vector Network Analyzer

1. Medical imaging

Medical imaging plays an important role in medical communication and education as well as research. X-ray, computed tomography (CT), ultrasound (US), magnetic resonance imaging (MRI), and positron emission tomography (PET) are most commonly used medical techniques. Most of them provide good resolution but each of them has some limitations. For example, X-ray can cause radiation, poses a health risk and it is less informative when it comes to imaging soft tissues. MRI is very expensive, further internal body movements such as heartbeat can produce measurement artifacts in an MRI image. Moreover, there may also be a chance of a false alarm when using these imaging techniques for tumor detection. This chapter reviews the existing medical imaging techniques, applications and limitations.

1.1 X-ray imaging and mammography

In 1895, Wilhelm Conrad Röntgen first discovered X-rays which caused worldwide excitement, especially in the medical field (Assmus, 1995). X-rays are generated in an X-ray tube by bombarding a heavy metal target with high-speed electrons and images are produced by passing the resulting radiation through the patient's body on to a photographic plate or digital recorder to produce a radiography, or by rotating both source and detector around the patient's body to produce a "slice" image by CT (Haidekker, 2013).

During X-ray measurement, patients are normally required to stand in front of a machine and press their bodies (image part) against a photographic plate. The technologist then activates the machine, which sends a beam of X-rays through. Patients are required to take deep breath and hold breath when they take chest or abdomen X-rays, these can help to reduce the chances of a blurred image. Although X-ray is a safe and painless procedure, it is also required to take special cares for patents by using the correct X-ray beam energies to ensure maximum safety. If an abnormality is found, additional imaging tests may be required, such as CT/MRI which is helpful in creating a more detailed picture of tissues, organs, and joints. Examples of specialized X-rays include angiograms, barium X-rays, and fluoroscopy.

X-ray mammography has been considered as the gold standard screening tool for early breast cancer detection, detecting about 75%

of cancers at least a year before they can be felt (Kamal et al., 2007). Mammography uses low dose X-rays, achieved by using targets made of low atomic weight alloys (e.g., molybdenum and rhodium). Mammography examinations consist of screening and diagnostic. Women beginning at 40 years of age are recommended to take mammography every year by the American Cancer Society, the American College of Radiology, the American College of Surgeons, and the American Congress of Obstetrics and Gynecology (Sadigh et al., 2011). Screening mammography may be performed as early as 25 years old in some patients with a very high lifetime risk of cancer (>20%) (Dorria Saleh et al., 2013). Studies have shown that regular mammograms may reduce the risk of late stage breast cancer in women 80 years of age and older (Badgwell et al., 2008).

Screening mammography should be based on age, family history of breast cancer, breast density, history of breast biopsy, and beliefs about the benefits and risks of the screening (Keen, 2008). Limitations include radiation, relatively high false negative rate (4% to 34%) (Huynh et al., 1998) and high false positive rate (70%) (Elmore et al., 1998), particularly with patients having dense breast tissue (Jackson et al., 1993). Detection is challenging for dense breast tissues (such as younger women) because there is less variation between the contrast of malignant and healthy tissues at X-ray frequencies. For example, younger women who normally presents a higher dense-to-fatty tissue ratio and lesions occurring in dense-tissue breasts are statistically more likely to be missed by X-ray mammography (Martin et al., 2009). Moreover, it is discomfort and pain due to breast compression that is required to reduce image blurring and to create uniform tissue density.

In factor, X-ray mammography appears to have reduced cancer death rates by only 0.0004%, which means it is not only unsafe but also not saving women's lives as was commonly thought (Smart, 1997). Research also showed that adding an annual mammogram to a careful physical examination of the breasts does not improve breast cancer survival rates over physical examination alone.

1.2 Computed tomography

In 1917, Radon reported computed tomography (CT) technique where the computer is essential in the image reconstruction (Radon, 1917). CT uses X-rays to create pictures of cross-sections of the body. During the exam, clinicians ask patients to lie on an examination table that slides into the center of the CT scanner. X-ray beam within the CT machine rotates around the body once the patient is inside the scanner. A computer creates separate images of the body, called slices. These images can be stored, viewed on a monitor, or printed on film. The patient is required to stay still during the exam to avoid blurred images which are caused by movement. He/she may be asked to hold his/her breath for short periods of time. Both 2D and 3D images can be generated by using CT scanner, 3D image of the body is created by stacking the slices together. Complete scans most often take only a few minutes. Modern clinical CT scanners are very fast, can perform the exam without stopping and can produce a 2D cross-sectional image in less than a second.

CT vastly exceeds projection X-ray imaging in soft tissue contrast, but the spatial resolution of a clinical whole-body CT scanner is lower than that of plain X-ray imaging. Nonetheless, CT can reveal small tumors, structural detail in trabecular bone or the alveolar tissue in the lungs. Spatial resolution can be as low as 100 μm in-plane, and specialized CT microscopes provide voxels of less than 10 μm. However, clinical CT scanners are expensive, ranging in the millions of dollars. This translates into a relatively high cost per CT scan, which prevents its more widespread adoption.

Certain CT exams require a special dye-contrast, to be delivered into the human body before the test starts. Contrast agents help certain areas show up better on the x-rays, it can be given several ways which depending on the type of CT being performed (Board, 2011). If contrast is required to use, a patient may be asked not to eat or drink anything for at least 4 hours before the test, normally a health care provider is referenced. Some people may feel uncomfortable due to lying on the hard table. Contrast given through a vein may cause a slight burning feeling, a metallic taste in the mouth, and a warm flushing of the body. These sensations are normal and usually go away within a few seconds.

CT scans have some limitations include allergic reaction to the contrast dye, damage to kidney function from the contrast dye and exposure. Compared to regular X-rays, CT scans expose more radiation. Taking many X-rays or CT scans in short period may increase the risk of cancer. The exam must be stopped immediately if any breathing problem occurs during the test.

1.3 Ultrasound

Ultrasound is one of the most widely used imaging technologies in medicine, which produces image based on the properties of sound waves in tissue (Chan et al., 2011). Pressure waves in the low megahertz range travel through tissue at the speed of sound, being refracted and partially reflected at interfaces. Ultrasound contrast is therefore related to echogenic in homogeneities in tissue. The depth of an echogenic object can be determined by the travel time of the echo. By emitting focused sound waves in different directions, 2D scans are possible. Ultrasound images are highly qualitative in nature due to the complex relationship between inhomogeneous tissue and the echoes, due to the differences in speed of sound in different tissues, and due to the high noise component that is a result of the weak signal and high amplification.

Ultrasound images present good soft tissue contrast, but fail in the presence of bone and air. Although ultrasound images can be generated with purely analog circuitry, modern ultrasound devices use computerized image processing for image formation, enhancement, and visualization. Ultrasound imaging is very popular because of its low-cost instrumentation and easy application. However, an ultrasound exam requires the presence of an experienced operator to adjust various parameters for optimum contrast, and ultrasound images usually require an experienced radiologist to interpret the image.

Ultrasound imaging involves the use of a small transducer and gel to expose the body and produces pictures of the inside of the body using high-frequency sound waves (Demi, 2014). The structure and movement of the body's internal organs as well as blood flowing through blood vessels can be identified in ultrasound images. It is able to differentiate skin, fat, glandular tissue and muscle in an ultrasound breast image. For women who are pregnant or at high risk for breast cancer and unable to undergo a mammography examination, may consider use ultrasound as a breast screening tool (Hou et al., 2002).

For early breast cancer detection, ultrasound can determine a breast cancer is a cyst or a lump, or a cyst with a lump inside, which is less efficient by X-ray inspection. However, it is impossible to identify many lesions by ultrasound imaging because the fat tissue has similar acoustic properties compared to cancer tissue. Another major limitation is the image quality highly depends on operator, this is because the procedures are performed using hand-held devices (Margarido et al., 2010).

1.4 Magnetic resonance imaging (MRI)

MRI image is generated based on the alignment change of hydrogen nuclei, which is caused by a magnetic field (generally 1.0T to 1.5T) and radio waves (Jacobs et al., 2007). A detailed MRI image allows physicians to evaluate various parts of human body and determine the presence of certain diseases. MRI has the ability to show dynamic functionality of the breast through the use of contrast agent injections. The main magnet, the gradient coils and the radiofrequency coils are the three major components of an MRI system. The sensitivity of MRI in visualizing invasive cancer is approximately 94% to 100% (Piccoli, 1997). Breast lesions can be detected successfully by using MRI while other medical imaging tools include mammogram failed (David et al., 2007). Recent research (Heil et al., 2012) reported that breast MRI increases the ability to detect small breast cancers in high-risk women compared to mammography and ultrasound. The impact of MRI on breast cancer recurrence or mortality, an analysis of the cost-effectiveness of MRI, optimize the application and performance of breast MRI, as well as clarify optimal acquisition protocols are significant works that need to be done in the future.

Similar to a certain extent CT, MRI is a volumetric imaging technique. But, the underlying physical principles are fundamentally different from CT (Haidekker, 2013). MRI is based on the orientation of protons inside a strong magnetic field, but CT uses high-energy photons and the interaction of photons with electrons of the atomic shell for contrast generation. This orientation can be manipulated with resonant radiofrequency waves, and the return of the protons to their equilibrium state can be measured. The relaxation time constants are highly tissue-dependent, and MRI features superior soft tissue contrast, by far exceeding that of CT.

Compared to CT, MRI normally requires longer time for image acquisition unless use special high-speed protocols. Modern MRI scanners require a superconductive magnet with liquid helium cooling infrastructure, extremely sensitive radiofrequency amplifiers, and a complete room shielded against electromagnetic interference. For this reason, MRI equipment is extremely expensive with costs of several million dollars for the scanner hardware and with accordingly high recurring costs for maintenance. However, MRI scanners provide images with a very high diagnostic value, and MRI can be used to monitor some physiological processes (e.g., water diffusion, blood oxygenation) and therefore partly overlaps with nuclear imaging modalities.

1.5 Trends in medical imaging technology

Table 1-1 compares the most available medical imaging techniques. X-ray imaging has reached a technological plateau. The trend moves toward digital X-ray imaging. Improved detectors with higher sensitivity allow to further reduce exposure time and the patient radiation dose. Use of X-rays in diagnostic and interventional procedures could lead to elevated cancer risk (Ron, 2003), therefore ultrasound and MRI techniques have received more attentions, which leading to a further reduction of the radiation exposure in patients.

CT is an attractive modality due to its very high per-slice acquisition rates, notably with the development of dual-source CT scanners (Davis et al., 1995). For example, the heart can be scanned in 3D during one heartbeat. In addition, modern CT scanners give rise to sub-mSv scans. Compared to 20 years ago, modern CT produces much less radiations.

Transmission-based X-ray imaging has recently been proposed by phase contrast and dark field methods that are known from light microscopy (Weitkamp, 2006). With suitable diffraction gratings, the phase can be converted into intensity and thus recorded by the detector (Pfeiffer et al., 2008). The same principle can be used to record scattered X-rays, leading to the X-ray analog of dark field imaging (Tilman et al., 2010). Phase contrast X-ray imaging provides the projection of the refractive index along the beam path, analogous to conventional X-ray imaging that provides the projection of the absorber density. Therefore, phase contrast-enhanced radiography advertises itself for CT reconstruction methods (Bech et al., 2010; Tilman et al., 2010). These methods promise not only markedly enhanced perception of contrast, but actually a different type of information retrieved from the scanned object, namely, its refractive index. Particularly in conjunction with CT reconstruction methods, tissue-tissue contrast could be dramatically enhanced, thus eliminating one weakness of X-ray based CT imaging.

Table 1-1 Comparison of existing medical imaging methods.

Method	X-ray mammography	CT	Ultrasound	MRI
Physical property	Tissue density	Tissue density	Tissue density	Hydrogen distribution and binding in tissues
Information provided	Structural includes micro-calcifications	Structural	Structural	Structural and functional
Spatial resolution	High	Low	Low	Low
Acquisition time	Seconds	Seconds	Minutes	Minutes
3D information	Yes	Yes	Yes	Yes
Anatomical distortion	Compression	Compression	Compression	Gravity
Issues	• Development of effective image processing; • Computer aided detection methods easily applied images; • Radiation;	• Allergic reaction to the contrast dye; • Damage to kidney function; radiation; • Increase the risk of cancer; • Radiation; • Expensive scanner;	• Less effective; • Too operator dependent; • Low contrast resolution;	• Magnetic coils and appropriate imaging sequence required; • Expensive method; • Proposed for staffing of cancer;

MRI experiences progress from the use of stronger magnets and improved amplifiers. Both lead to higher spatial resolution and improved signal noise ratio (SNR), or, with constant SNR, to shorter acquisition times (Andrew, 2012). Blood-oxygen level dependent (BOLD) sequence allows to measure blood flow and blood oxygenation levels (Ogawa et al., 1990). BOLD functional images are often superimposed over structural MRI images that have low SNR and lower spatial resolution. Another functional MRI should spend time to investigate is diffusion tensor imaging, which allows to recover the 3D vector field of water diffusion (Cercignani et al., 2001). Clinical applications can be brain imaging in dementia, including Alzheimer's disease (Bihan et al., 2001). Normally, MR is not widely popular for bone imaging due to the low proton density and the short relaxation times in bone (Magland et al., 2009). Micro-MRI imaging makes use of reduced T_2^* as a consequence of microscopic susceptibility changes caused by bone (Wehrli et al., 2002). Micro-MRI imaging of bone promises to evolve into one pillar of trabecular structure assessment (Haidekker et al., 2011).

Ultrasound imaging technology has also reached a certain plateau. It remains the modality of choice for rapid, low-cost diagnostic procedures without ionizing radiation. Over the last two decades, the size of ultrasound scanners were reduced dramatically, and recently hand-held ultrasound scanners with full diagnostic capabilities were proposed (Prinz et al., 2011). It is expected that the popularity of ultrasound imaging will further increase with the spread of ultra-portable devices. Ultrasound contrast agents were introduced that consist of gas-filled micro-bubbles. These bubbles literally burst in the incident sound field and create a strong signal. These micro-bubbles can be functionalized to bind to specific sites, such as tumors or inflammatory processes (Kiessling et al., 2012). Such contrast agents will help ultrasound move toward functional imaging, with the additional potential for targeted drug delivery (Ferrara et al., 2009) because the micro-bubbles can be loaded with drugs, set to burst at the insonicated target site.

1.6 Closure

Several existing medical imaging approaches include X-ray, CT, Ultrasound and MRI, their applications, limitations and trends in medical areas are reviewed in this Chapter. Although X-ray mammography remains the most commonly used technique, some limitations include inaccurate, uncomfortable due to breast compression, can provoke cancer due to ionizing radiation, is unusable during surgery and is relatively expensive. Ultrasound and MRI play important roles in breast cancer detection, however, they are either not yet sensitive enough, have low contrast resolution (small lesions are not detectable), less effective, too operator dependent, or too expensive for screening purpose. It is urgent to develop a new safe, low-cost, reliable technique to compliment X-ray mammography with high image contrast and resolution for early breast cancer detection. Microwave imaging has been proposed as one of the most promising emerging imaging technologies for breast cancer detection. The development of new approaches to overcome the current challenges of medical imaging techniques for breast lesion detection is needed. The next chapter introduces the microwave imaging approach and their applications in the medical field.

2. Microwave imaging

Microwave imaging techniques have shown good capabilities in various fields such as civil engineering, nondestructive testing, industrial applications, and have in recent decades experienced strong growth as a research topic in biomedical diagnostics. This chapter introduces and describes the concept of microwave imaging with some applications in the biomedical field.

2.1 Electrical properties of the tissue

In the 1970s, Larsen and Jacobi using microwave sensing and imaging technologies produced an image of canine kidney (Jacobi et al., 1978; Larsen et al., 1978). Since then using microwave sensing and imaging techniques for medical diagnosis have been investigated by many researchers worldwide. The working principle of microwave sensing and imaging for medical diagnosis is the different electrical properties between different tissues which can be measured and identified in an image. Different types of biological tissues have distinct electrical properties (relative permittivity and conductivity) due to differences in the water content (Schepps et al., 1980).

In 1989, Foster et al. reported a critical review of dielectric properties of human tissues (Foster et al., 1989). In 1994, Joines et al. measured the electrical properties of various healthy and the malignant tissues from 50 MHz to 900 MHz (Joines et al., 1994), their measurement results are shown in Figure 2-1. It is can be seen that the relative permittivity can either increase (for breast, colon, and liver) or can even decrease (for lung and kidney) for the malignant tissue. The increase was highest in the case of breast, whereas for the kidney, low difference was measured. For the conductivity (see Figure 2-1(b)), breast tissues have the biggest difference and kidney have the least difference.

In 1996, Gabriel reported the dielectric properties measurements of various healthy tissues (Gabriel et al., 1996a; Gabriel et al., 1996b). Lazebnik measured the dielectric properties of normal breast and cancerous tissues in the frequency range 0.5 GHz to 20 GHz (Lazebnik et al., 2007a). Figure 2-2 shows the dielectric properties of normal breast tissues having a wide range of values depending on tissue type. Results illustrated that both the dielectric constant and conductivity tend to decrease as the adipose content increases, and conversely as the percentage

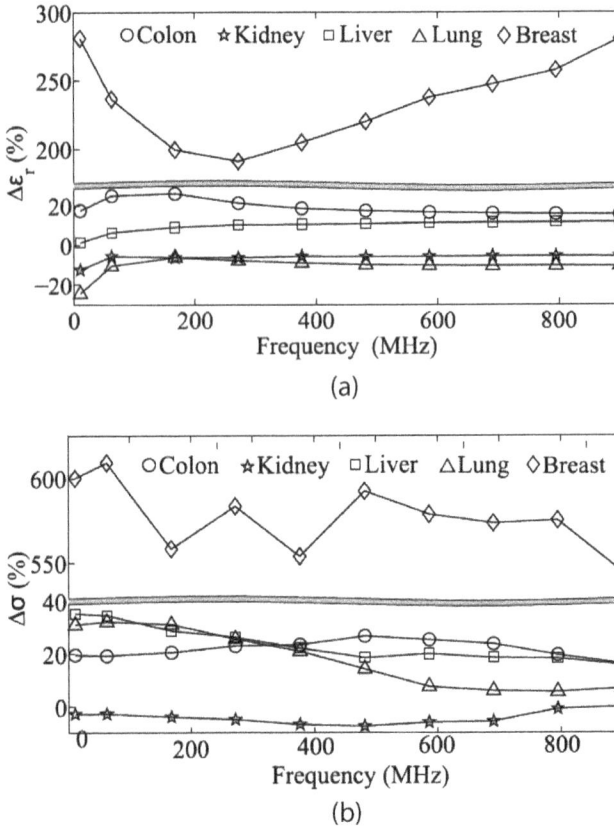

Figure 2-1   Percentage change in the electrical properties of malignant tissues with respect to the healthy tissue from 50 to 900 MHz: (a) percentage change in the relative permittivity (b) percentage change in the conductivity (Joines et al., 1994).

of glandular and/or fibro-connective tissue increases, both the dielectric constant and conductivity increase (Lazebnik et al., 2007b).

The electrical properties of various biological tissues, including heart for myocardial ischemia and infarction (Semenov et al., 1996; Semenov et al., 2000), skin (Sunaga et al., 2002), liver (O'Rourke et al., 2007), breast tissues (Bindu et al., 2007; Lazebnik et al., 2007; Ryan et al., 2009), bone (Meaney et al., 2012) and lymph nodes (Deighton, 2013), have been investigated by many researchers. A variety of factors have been explored and explains the difference in electrical properties between healthy and malignant tissues include water content (Schepps et al., 1980), charging of the cell membrane (Pethig, 1984), difference

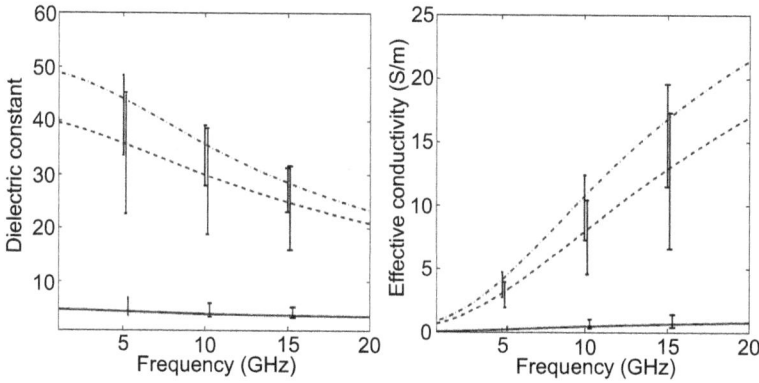

Figure 2-2 Measured dielectric properties of the three tissue groups defined by percentage adipose tissue present in the sample. The variability bars show the 25th–75th percentiles of the fitted values. Dash-dot line: group 1 (0% to 30% adipose), dashed line: group 2 (31% to 84% adipose), solid line: group 3 (85% to 100% adipose) (Lazebnik et al., 2007b).

in the sodium content (Pethig, 1984), necrosis and inflammation causing breakdown of cell membrane (Sha et al., 2002), and change in the dielectric relaxation time (Lazebnik et al., 2007).

2.2 Model of the electrical properties of biological tissue

In biological tissues, both the dielectric permittivity and conductivity are strongly non-linear functions of frequency (Joines et al., 1994). Choose suitable frequency range is a critical task for imaging because the attenuation of the microwave signal increases with the frequency due to increase in the conductivity resulting in a lower penetration depth. Various models have been developed to model the frequency dispersive nature of the tissue, where the two most commonly used models are the Debye model and the Cole-Cole model (Gabriel et al., 1996b). The Debye model sufficiently models the frequency dependence of the complex permittivity of the tissues, and this model is defined as (Andreas et al., 2012):

$$\varepsilon_r = \varepsilon_\infty + \frac{\varepsilon_s + \varepsilon_\infty}{1 + j\omega\tau} - j\frac{\sigma}{\omega\varepsilon_0} \qquad (2\text{-}1)$$

Where
ε_∞ = permittivity value of the tissue
ε_s = static permittivity of the tissue

ε_0 = permittivity of free-space
τ = characteristic relaxation time of the medium
σ = conductivity of the tissue
ω = angle frequency

Cole-Cole model was proposed by K. S. Cole and R. H. Cole (Said et al., 2009):

$$\varepsilon^*(\omega) = \varepsilon_\infty + \frac{\varepsilon_s - \varepsilon_\infty}{1 + (j\omega\tau)^{1-\alpha}} \qquad (2\text{-}2)$$

Where ε^* is the complex dielectric constant, ε_s and ε_∞ are static and infinite frequency dielectric constants, ω is the angular frequency and τ is a time constant. The exponent parameter α, which takes a value between 0 and 1 describes different spectral shapes. When $\alpha = 0$, the Cole-Cole model reduces to the Debye model. When $\alpha > 0$, the relaxation is stretched.

2.3 Imaging methods

As shown in Figure 2-3, when an dielectric object (lesion) with contrast in the constitutive parameters, ε_{obj}, and conductivity, σ_{obj}, is positioned inside a microwave imaging system, a scattered field will arise. The total field can be defined as:

$$E_{tot} = E_{inc} + E_{scat} \qquad (2\text{-}3)$$

Where E_{inc} is the incident field and E_{scat} is the backscattered field.

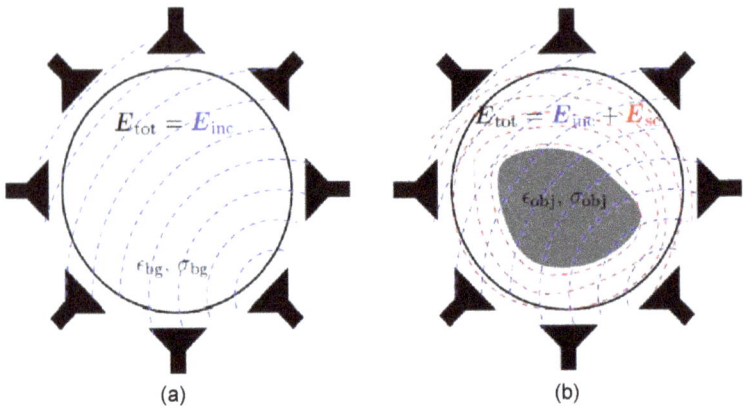

(a)   (b)

Figure 2-3 Schematic of a microwave imaging system (a) empty system (b) object inserted in system (Rubæk, 2008).

Several microwave imaging systems were developed to measure the backscattered field and to generate images of dielectric objects. There are three main microwave imaging approaches: Hybrids, passive and active microwave imaging techniques. Hybrid approaches using microwave signals to heat tissues and comparing the differential pressure waves generated by the mechanical expansion of the tissues to detect lesions. Passive microwave using radiometric techniques to measure temperature differences between normal and malignant tissues and identify the lesions based on the measurement differences.

Active microwave imaging techniques generate microwave signals into the target objects and measure the reflections from the objects by employing a set of receivers or by recording the reflections at the transmitter antenna (Ibrahim et al., 2008). Two main active microwave imaging approaches are microwave tomography (Semenov, 2009) and radar-based imaging (Li et al., 2001; Kurrant et al., 2008). Different tomographic techniques (Semenov et al., 1996; Colin et al., 2001; Epstein et al., 2014) have been suggested for imaging of the breast, such as single-frequency, multi-frequency, and time-domain tomography. These algorithms have different requirements to the hardware of the imaging system as well as the computational power needed to create the images.

Three major radar-based microwave imaging techniques are microwave imaging via space time (MIST) (Li et al., 2004), tissue sensing adaptive radar (TSAR) system (Fear et al., 2002) and indirect holographic technique (Smith et al., 2014). Hagness proposed confocal microwave imaging approach, which aims to identify the presence and location of strong scattered reflections based on the significant contrast between the lesion and healthy breast tissues (Hagness et al., 1998). This technology could provide both the necessary imaging resolution and penetration depth in the breast. The patient lies in a supine position during operation. Seventeen receivers were used to record the reflections, and a spherical lesion of 5 mm diameter that was located 3 cm beneath the array was detected successfully. In their 3D study (Hagness et al., 1999), a resistively loaded 8 cm long bowtie antenna was used as a sensor and a circular lesion of 1.76 cm diameter located 5 cm below the antenna was detected. However, this approach does not compensate for frequency-dependent propagation effects and has limited ability to discriminate against artifacts and noise.

MIST system was developed by Bond (Bond et al., 2003), in which the beam former spatially focuses the backscattered signals to discriminate against clutter and noise while compensating for frequency-dependent propagation effects. During an operation, the patient was lying in a supine (face-up) position on the examination table with the antennas scanned over the naturally flattened breast. The simulation results showed that a 2 mm lesion in a 2D breast model derived from magnetic resonance imaging could be detected. The same researcher group also developed a method to remove skin-breast interface that produced artifacts in the image prior to performing lesion detection. In 2004 (Li et al., 2004) they presented an experimental setup consisting of a breast phantom simulated as a container filled with a liquid mimicking normal breast tissue, a small synthetic lesion suspended in the liquid and a thin layer of material representing the skin layer.

Fear's group developed TSAR system (Fear et al., 2002). During an operation, the patient was lying in the prone position on the examination table with her breast extending through a hole in the examination table and the antennas were scanned around the breast. The image algorithm requires three steps, first place the tissue sensing to locate the breast in the tank, the skin reflections are estimated and subtracted and finally the breast image is formed from the reflection signals without skin reflections. The TSAR technique has the ability to detect and localize lesions (>4 mm diameter). Difficulties of such a technique include large reflections from the skin and expensive ultra-high speed digital electronics for real-time imaging.

Indirect holography microwave (IHM) involves recording of a holographic intensity pattern and reconstructing the image by using Fourier transformation from the 2D holographic intensity pattern produced (Smith et al., 2004). Compared to TSAR technique, IHM does not require expensive ultra-high speed electronics, as narrow-band signals can be converted to the broadband for digitization at a slower rate, thereby enabling real-time imaging at a lower cost. It offers high contrast between healthy and malignant tissues and assists in forming an image of the location and extent of the malignant tissue.

2.4 Development of microwave imaging systems

Microwave measurement system plays an important role in a microwave imaging system, which normally contains a microwave signal transmitter and a receiver such as a vector network analyzer, an antenna array, and a radio frequency switch that switches between different antennas (Henriksson et al., 2001). Several experimental setups were developed for imaging of microwave biological objects as shown in Table 2-1.

The measurements conducted by Larsen and Jacobi using a developed antenna which was immersed in water (Larsen et al., 1986). The major limitation of such system is the long acquisition time required. Further, this early work used intensity modulation of a raster scanned display to convert measured scattering parameters into an image.

As shown in Figure 2-4, an array of antennas encircling the breast phantom were proposed by Fear (Fear et al., 2000), both the array and the breast were immersed in matching mediums, one medium with

Table 2-1 Experimental microwave imaging systems.

	Dartmouth College (USA)	Keele University (UK)	University of Bristol (UK)	University of Manitoba (Canada)
Antenna	Circular array of 16 monopoles	Circular array of 24 ceramic filled opened waveguides	Two spherical arrays consist of 31 and 60 ultra-wideband antennas	Circular array of doubled layers Vivaldy antennas
Frequency	0.5~3 GHz	1.0~2.3 GHz	4–8 GHz	3–6 GHz
Test phantom	Real patients	Soft animal tissues	Real breasts	Various dielectric objects
Immersion medium	0.9% saline ($\varepsilon_r = 76.6$, $\sigma = 2.48$ S/m)	Metallic bath with coupling liquid	Matching ceramic	No matching medium, air only
Image	2D and 3D	2D	3D	2D
Clinical trial	Yes	No	Yes	No

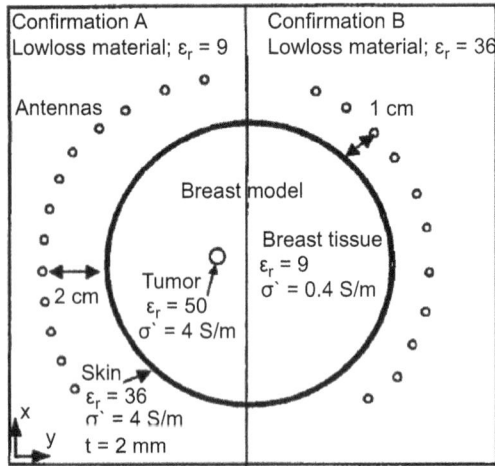

Figure 2-4 System configurations when the antenna array is immersed in coupling medium (Fear et al., 2000).

dielectric properties close to breast tissue and one medium with properties close to that of the skin. The experiments resulted in successful detection for both couplings; however, the second matching medium showed an increased sensitivity to the presence of a tumor. Dipole antenna was used in her study due to its small size and low cost with reasonable bandwidth. However, such antenna has low efficiency and directivity.

In 2002, Fear's group proposed a confocal microwave imaging system (Fear et al., 2002) that contains a cylindrical array of loaded dipole antennas. A hemispherical realistic breast phantom, using MRI technique was developed, which includes a more glandular structure, nipple, skin, normal tissue, chest wall and tumor (see Figure 2-5).

In 2003, Hagness's group developed a microwave imaging via space-time (MIST) system (Li et al., 2003). Figure 2-6 shows an experimental setup of a planar microwave imaging system. A planar array of ultra-wideband (UWB) horn antennas was used to transmit microwave signals into the breast phantom and to receive signals from several antenna locations. To remove skin-breast interface that produced artifacts in the image prior, they developed a new method to performing lesion detection. In 2004, they presented an experimental system that consists of a breast phantom simulated as a container filled with a liquid mimicking normal breast tissue, a small synthetic lesion suspended in the liquid and a thin layer of material representing the skin layer (Li et al., 2004).

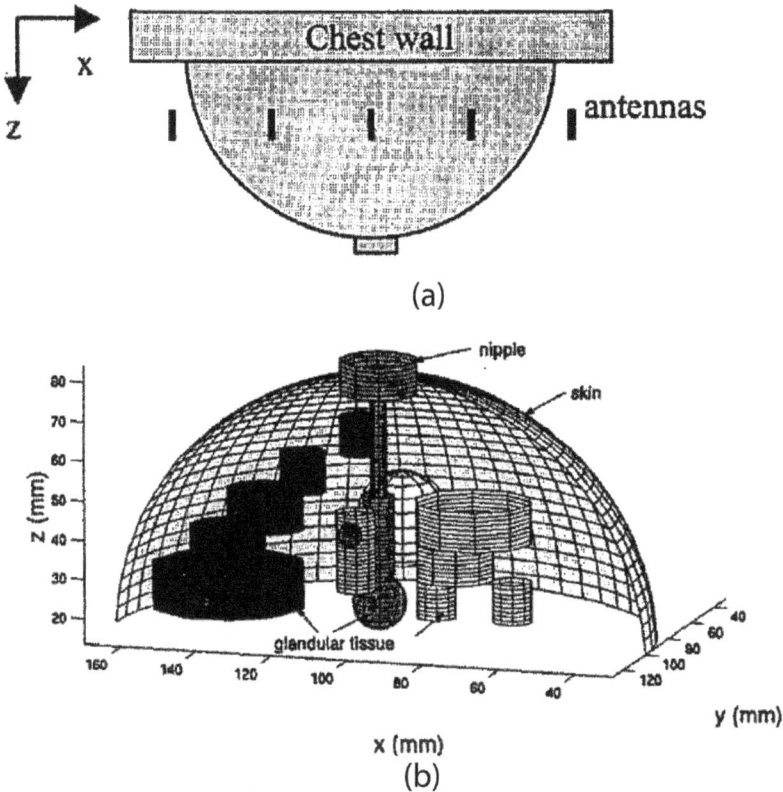

(a)

(b)

Figure 2-5 The hemispherical breast model (a) The orientations of the chest wall and antenna locations are indicated. (b) The interior of the model contains objects representing glandular tissue (Fear et al., 2002).

In 2006, researchers at University of Bristol developed a microwave imaging measurement system using hemi-spherical conformal array over the frequency range from 4 GHz to 10 GHz (see Figure 2-7), and the designed system was evaluated on a breast phantom (Figure 2-8). They found that improving the bandwidth of the array element may improve the image quality (Craddock et al., 2006).

In 2007, researchers at Dartmouth College developed a microwave tomography imaging system for clinical trial over the frequency range from 500 MHz to 3 GHz (see Figure 2-9). The system contains a cylindrical array of sixteen monopole antennas, where one used as transmitter and others as receivers, to transmit microwave signals into dielectric

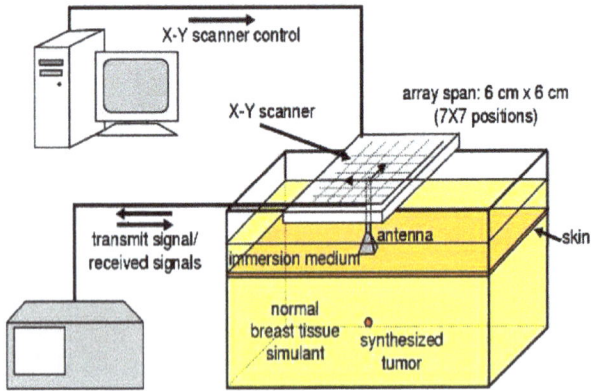

Figure 2-6 Experimental setup of a planar microwave imaging system (Li et al., 2004).

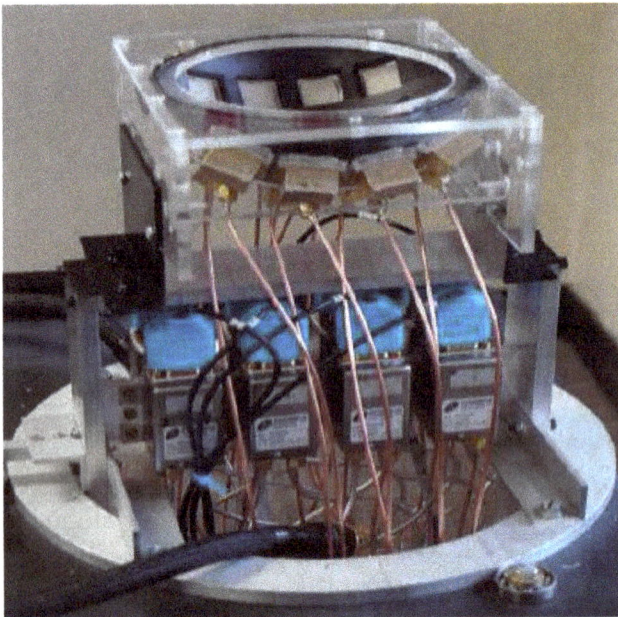

Figure 2-7 University of Bristol's conformal array experimental setup (Craddock et al., 2006).

objects and measure the scattered signals from the objects. The dielectric permittivity of the coupling medium was close to fatty tissues. This system was validated on breast phantoms and real human subjects, results demonstrated the possibility of using microwave imaging to detect breast cancer clinically (Meaney et al., 2007).

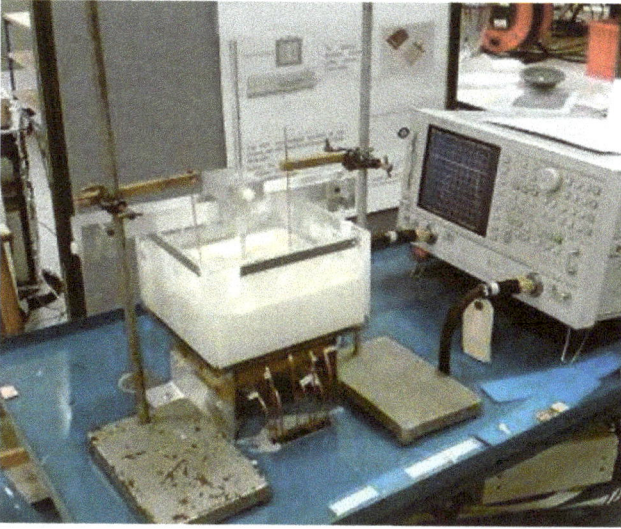

Figure 2-8 University of Bristol's phantom-based experimental setup (Craddock et al., 2006).

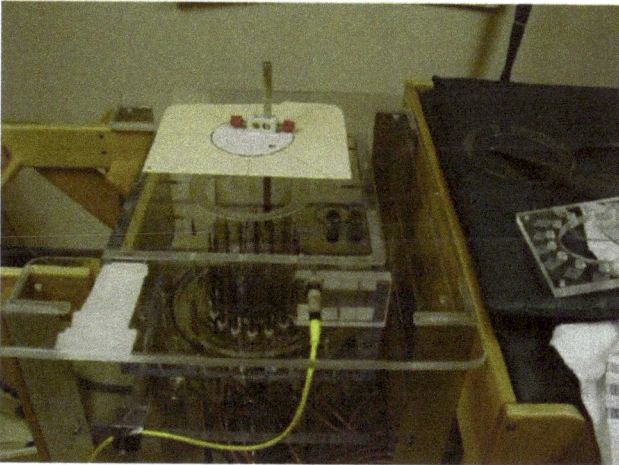

Figure 2-9 Dartmouth College's microwave imaging system (Meaney et al., 2007).

In 2011, an UWB cylindrical microwave imaging system was developed as shown in Figure 2-10, it incorporating a circular scanning system with the ability to mechanically rotate the sub-system in order to obtain more scanning angles (Marek et al., 2010). The system contains a tapered slot antenna and a breast phantom. The breast phantom

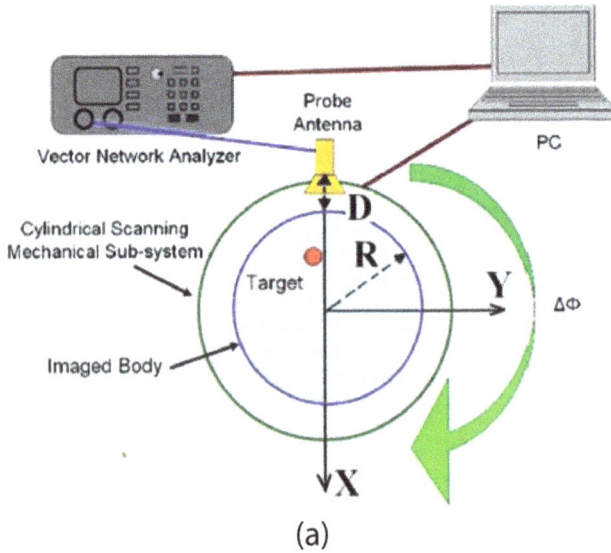

(a)

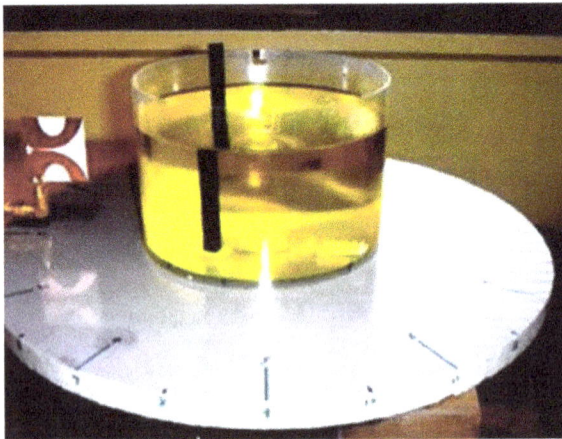

(b)

Figure 2-10 (a) Configuration of microwave imaging system; (b) Photograph of an imaged body with a target illuminated by a tapered slot (Marek et al., 2010).

consisted of a cylindrical container filled with oil to represent the fat tissue and a small plastic circular cylinder filled with water to represent the tumor.

In 2012, John's group (John et al., 2012) developed a prototype microwave imaging system incorporating an integrated numerical characterization technique. The system consists of an imaging cavity formed from 12 panels soldered together and each panel includes 3 bow-tie antennas (see Figure 2-11(a)). Figure 2-11(b) shows the experimental setup of the system, in which the imaging cavity was connected to the vector network analyzer through a solid-state switching

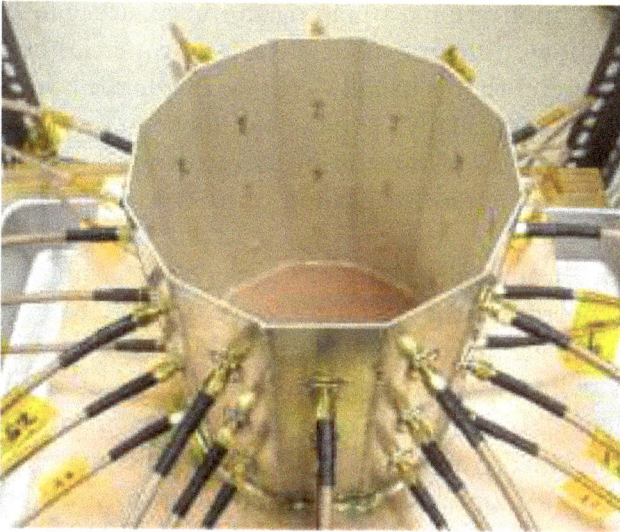

(a)

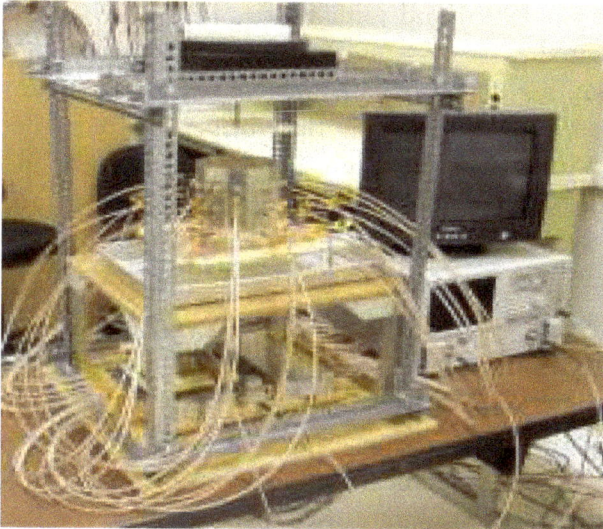

(b)

Figure 2-11 (a) Imaging cavity; (b) Experimental setup (John et al., 2012).

matrix. In order to obtain a multiple transmitter viewer, the rotators were mounted and turned the suspended objects. The cavity was filled in a coupling medium, and an image of a spherical object was reconstructed by using inverse scattering algorithm.

2.5 Microwave imaging applications

In the imaging applications, a map or an image either in 2D or 3D is formed, that shows different tissue electrical properties or the location of a strong scatterer that is usually a tumor inside the body. Microwave imaging systems are usually portable and low cost, and hence, can offer the initial diagnosis of various life threatening conditions like brain strokes while patients are still being on the way to a hospital in an ambulance.

Various medical applications of microwave sensing and imaging have been reported in the literature. Several data acquisition setups, including linear arrangements of antennas (Pichot et al., 1985) and much faster cylindrical arrangements (Broquetas et al., 1991), have been investigated. Investigation of microwave imaging has moved from simple imaging of organs to applications specific imaging for various pathological conditions. Various applications include breast image (Nikolova, 2011), bone imaging (Meaney et al., 2012), heart imaging (Semenov et al., 1996) and joint tissues (Salvador et al., 2010) have been investigated.

Initial study for detection of multiple lymph nodes in the axillary region using microwave Imaging have been reported (Eleuterio et al., 2015), which caused worldwide excitement, especially in the medical imaging field. Nikolova (Nikolova, 2011) and Fear et al. (Fear et al., 2002) have extensively reviewed the research work done for breast cancer imaging. Microwave sensing and imaging technique is emerging as a low cost and low health risk alternative to existing medical imaging techniques.

2.6 Challenges and future works

Many promising indicators suggested that microwave systems in the future will be a successful clinical complement to conventional mammography. However, existing microwave measurement systems have some limitations. The phantoms used in the measurement systems developed to date consist of either a simple mixture or simple materials to represent the human tissues. Some challenges toward practical implement of microwave imaging techniques caused due to the electrical properties difference between the normal and the malignant tissue might be lower than people thought. Further, the presence of multiple tissues with different properties results in a complex scattering environment. The frequency dispersion of electrical properties of the tissues that results in the distortion of the wideband pulses is another challenge. These challenges can be solved by developing a high dynamic system to capture the small difference in the scattered field or develop a contrast agent to enhance the electrical properties of the malignant tissues.

2.7 Closure

Several microwave imaging approaches and prototype systems were presented in this chapter. Various medical applications of the microwave sensing and imaging techniques were demonstrated. The development of new approaches to overcome the current limitations of microwave imaging techniques for tumor detection in particular in breast lesion is needed. The next chapter introduces the proposed new microwave imaging approach.

3. Principles of holographic microwave imaging

This chapter presents an initial analysis and development of holographic microwave imaging (HMI) techniques. This study starts with developing a 2D imaging model in a 3D geometry system in order to save computation time and easily investigate the proposed technique.

3.1 Introduction

The idea of the HMI technique for imaging of dielectric object is based on the holographic and aperture synthesis far-field imaging technique similar to the one widely used in radio astronomy. The process involves transmitting microwave signals to a dielectric object by a single transmitting antenna and measuring the backscattered electric field from a dielectric object by an array of antennas and using image processing algorithms on the measured data to reconstruct an image.

3.2 2D imaging algorithm development

Figure 3-1 shows a block diagram of a HMI technique. A 3D geometry relevant to the HMI technique is show in Figure 3-2, where x, y and z

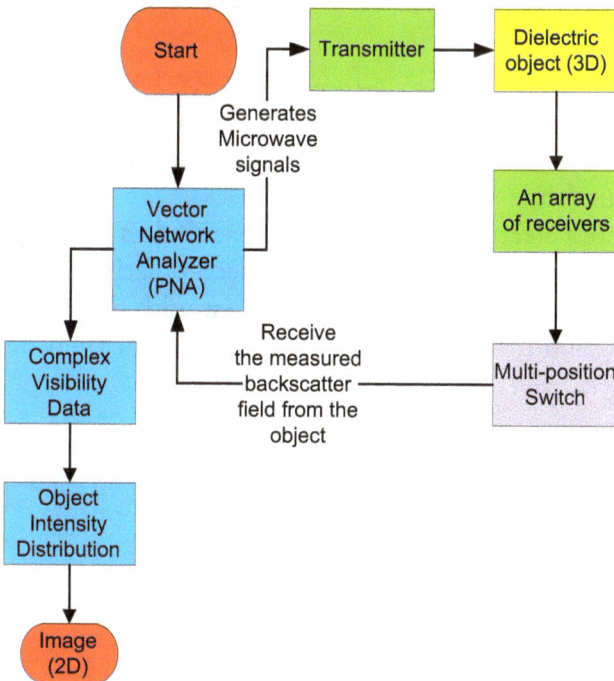

Figure 3-1　The block diagram of 3D HMI technique setup.

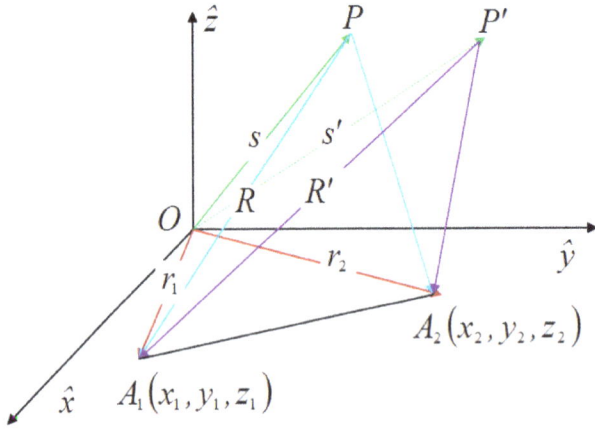

Figure 3-2 Geometry of HMI measurements by a pair of antennas.

represent antenna locations in the array plane. A point $P(x', y', z')$ was assumed as a point in a dielectric object, under far-field conditions the visibility function **G** of the backscattered electric field E_{scat} for any two antennas located at r_1 and r_2 was defined as (Levanda et al., 2010):

$$G(r_1, r_2) = <E_{scat}(r_1) \cdot E_{scat}^*(r_2)>$$ (3-1)

Where the asterisk denotes the complex conjugate and stands for the expected value (time average).

The scattered electric field can be represented as an integral over the volume of the scatterer involving the induced polarisation currents that arise from the complex permittivity contrast with the host medium. In the far-field condition, the backscattered field can then be written as follows (Silver, 1984):

$$E_{scat}(r) = \left(\frac{k_0^2}{4\pi}\right) \int_V (\varepsilon(s) - \varepsilon_b) E_T(s) \frac{e^{-jk_b|s-r|}}{|s-r|} dV$$ (3-2)

Where
$j = \sqrt{-1}$,
$k_0 = 2\pi/\lambda_0$,
$k_b = 2\pi/\lambda_b$,

λ_0 = Wavelength in free space,
λ_b = Wavelength in host medium,
$\varepsilon(s)$ = Complex relative permittivity distribution of object,
ε_b = Complex relative permittivity of host medium,
r = Position vector from a point in the breast to the receiving antenna,
$E_T(s)$ = Total electric field (incident plus scattered) at a point inside the dielectric object with position vector s.

Substituting for the scattered fields in Equation (3-1) using Equation (3-2) gives the following six-fold integral for the complex visibility function:

$$G(r_1, r_2) = \left(\frac{k_0^2}{4\pi} \right)^2 \iiint_V \iiint_{V'} (\varepsilon(s) - \varepsilon_b)(\varepsilon(s') - \varepsilon_b)^* \quad (3\text{-}3)$$

$$E_T(s) \cdot E_T^*(s') \frac{e^{-jk_b(R-R')}}{RR'} dVdV'$$

Where $R = |r_1 - s|$ and $R' = |r_1 - s'|$.
If the distance from a point P to the receiving antenna A_1 is very large compared to the size of antenna array plane, which is $R \gg |r_1|$ then:

$$R = |R| = \sqrt{(r_1 - s) \cdot (r_1 - s)} = \sqrt{r_1^2 + s^2 - 2r_1 \cdot s} \quad (3\text{-}4)$$

$$\cong s - \frac{r_1 \cdot s}{s} = s - r_1 \cdot \hat{s}$$

Where the "dot" denotes the scalar product and $\hat{s}$ is a unit vector. Similarly, the distance from another point P' within the object to the receiving antenna can be calculated as:

$$R' = |R'| = s' - r_2 \cdot \hat{s'} \quad (3\text{-}5)$$

Then

$$\frac{e^{-jk_b(R-R')}}{RR'} \approx \frac{1}{ss'} e^{-jk_b(s-s')} e^{jk_b(r_2\hat{s'} - r_1\hat{s})} \quad (3\text{-}6)$$

The six-fold integral of Equation (3-3) can be simplified by noting that the phase factor $e^{-jk_b(s-s')}$ oscillates rapidly as the operator scans over all possible pairs of points (P, P') within the domain of integration. Consequently, the only significant contribution to the value of the integral in Equation (3-3) arises from points for which the phase varies slowly. This situation corresponds to the case for which the points (P, P') coincide. Therefore, $s - s' \to 0$ is allowed, so that $s - s'$.

The visibility function where the integration is over the volume of the dielectric object can be obtained:

$$G(r_1, r_2) = \left(\frac{k_0^2}{4\pi} \right)^2 \iiint_V (|\mathcal{E}(s) - \mathcal{E}_b|^2)$$

(3-7)

$$E_T(s) \cdot E_T^*(s') \frac{e^{-jk_b(r_1 - r_2')\cdot \hat{s}}}{s^2} dV$$

Defining the object intensity function at the position s as:

$$I(s) = \left(\frac{k_0^2}{4\pi} \right)^2 |\mathcal{E}(s) - \mathcal{E}_b|^2 E_T(s) \cdot E_T^*(s)$$

(3-8)

The baseline vector can be defined as:

$$D = (r_1 - r_2)/\lambda_b$$

(3-9)

Equation (3-7) can be rewritten as:

$$G(D) = \iiint_V I(s) \frac{e^{-j2\pi D \cdot s}}{s^2} dV$$

(3-10)

Let the Cartesian components of the unit vector $\hat{s}$ be expressed in spherical polar coordinates (θ, ϕ) as follows (see Figure 3-3):

$$\hat{s} = \sin\theta \cos\phi \hat{x} + \sin\theta \sin\phi \hat{y} + \cos\theta \hat{z}$$

(3-11)

The volume element dV becomes:

$$dV = s^2 \sin\theta d\theta d\phi ds$$

(3-12)

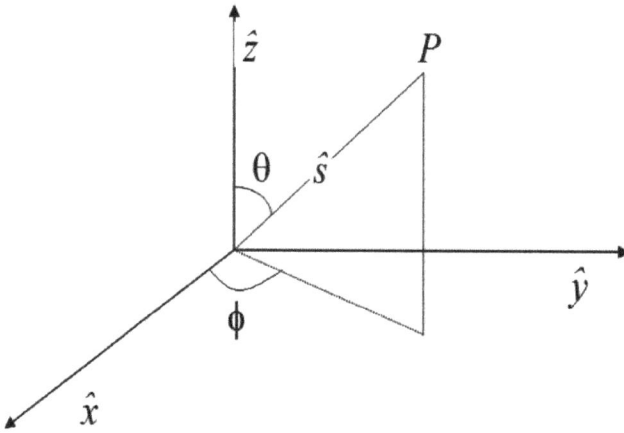

Figure 3-3   Spherical polar coordinate system.

Defining new variables (l, m, n) as:

$$l = \sin\theta\cos\phi$$
$$m = \sin\theta\sin\phi \qquad (3\text{-}13)$$
$$n = \cos\theta = \sqrt{1 - l^2 - m^2}$$

The element dV can be written as:

$$dV = s^2 dl\,dm\,ds/n \qquad (3\text{-}14)$$

Substituting Equation (3-14) into Equation (3-10), a more useful form can be obtained:

$$G(\mathbf{D}) = \iiint_V I(s)\frac{e^{-j2\pi \mathbf{D}\cdot\hat{s}}}{n} dl\,dm\,ds \qquad (3\text{-}15)$$

Writing the Cartesian components of the baseline vector $\mathbf{D}$ as (u, v, w) such that:

$$u = (x_2 - x_1)/\lambda_b$$
$$v = (y_2 - y_1)/\lambda_b \qquad (3\text{-}16)$$
$$w = (z_2 - z_1)/\lambda_b$$

The visibility function then can be defined as:

$$G(u,v,w) = \int_l \int_m \int_s \frac{I(s,l,m)}{\sqrt{1-l^2-m^2}} e^{-j2\pi\Phi} dl\, dm\, ds \qquad (3\text{-}17)$$

Where $\Phi = D \cdot \hat{s} = ul + vm + wn$

All antennas were assumed to be located on a 2D plane then $w = 0$. A line integral along the radial coordinate s was defined as:

$$\tilde{I}(l,m) = \int_s \frac{I(s,l,m)}{\sqrt{1-l^2-m^2}} ds \qquad (3\text{-}18)$$

Then a 2D visibility function was developed using Equation (3-18):

$$G(u,v,0) = \int\int \tilde{I}(l,m)e^{-j2\pi(ul+vm)} dl\, dm \qquad (3\text{-}19)$$

It is can be seen that the visibility function is a 2D Fourier transform of the 2D intensity function $\tilde{I}(l,m)$, which was consistent with the Van Cittert-Zernike theorem (Born et al., 1980). Therefore, the 2D intensity function was defined by inverse Fourier transform:

$$\tilde{I}(l,m) = \int\int G(u,v,0)e^{j2\pi(ul+vm)} du\, dv \qquad (3\text{-}20)$$

Equation (3-20) presents if measurements of the visibility function $G(u,v)$ that span the space (u,v) are available then a 2D image can be determined by using an inverse Fourier transform. The 2D image generated by using the intensity function $\tilde{I}(l,m)$ was defined by the line integral in Equation (3-18) and represents the scattering intensity in the object integrated along each radial vector.

3.3 3D imaging algorithm development

To obtain a 3D image, a 3D dielectric object was assumed contains multi-layers. The antenna array plane was designed to be moveable from H_1(mm) to H_n(mm) in equal M steps, where H is the distance between antenna array plane and the model (see Figure 3-4). Then the lesion at depth location z_n within the same object was defined as:

$$z_n = s_n \cos(\theta_n) \qquad (3\text{-}21)$$

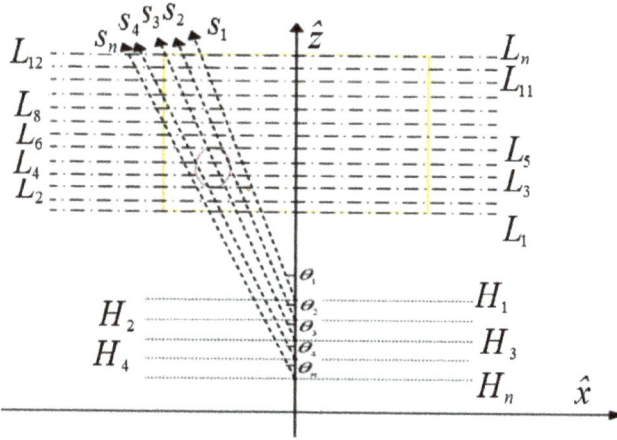

Figure 3-4 Block diagram showing the scattering characterization scheme from different receiving height H_n.

Where θ_n is the transmitting or receiving angle of the same antenna on the antenna array plane to the detected object at the position s_n with the antenna array plane to model at the distance H_n.

Thus ds in Equation (3-18) became:

$$ds = \frac{dz}{\cos(\theta_n)} = \frac{dz}{\sqrt{1-l^2-m^2}} \qquad (3\text{-}22)$$

By differentiating Equation (3-18), the 3D image of the object intensity function at a selected height $H = H_n$, can be obtained.

$$I(H=z_n,l,m) = \frac{d\tilde{I}(l,m)\cdot(1-l^2-m^2)}{dz} \qquad (3\text{-}23)$$

The derivative in Equation (3-23) can be approximated by the following forward difference expression:

$$\frac{d\tilde{I}}{dz} = \frac{\tilde{I}_{z_n}-\tilde{I}_{z_{n-1}}}{z_n-z_{n-1}} \qquad (3\text{-}24)$$

A reconstructed 3D image of the object intensity function was then computed using Equation (3-23) and Equation (3-24) by placing the antenna array plane at difference heights. To quantitatively assess imaging results, a zooming function can be applied to enhance the image contrast:

$$\tilde{I}_m(H,l,m) = [\tilde{I}(H,l,m)]^{\mathcal{Q}} \qquad (3\text{-}25)$$

Equation (3-25) performs a zoom on an image of the object.

3.4   Closure

The complex visibility function was computed by using Equation (3-1) for all possible pairs of receivers, with the background scattered field subtracted from the data. For example, for N receivers, the measured complex visibility data is $N(N-1)$. Referring to Equation (3-1) and Equation (3-20), a 2D image can be represented by using complex visibility data that was collected when the antenna array plane was placed at a selected height. A reconstructed 3D image of the object was computed using Equation (3-23) and Equation (3-24) by acquiring measured data with the antenna array placed at different heights, and computing the sequence of 2D images $\tilde{I}_{Z_n}$. Next chapter presents the experimental validation of the proposed technique.

4. Measurement system of holographic microwave imaging

This chapter presents the experimental measurement setups of the proposed technique for diagnosing inclusions within dielectric objects, and in particular, it relates to electromagnetic imaging to reconstruct dielectric properties of inhomogeneous, lossy bodies with arbitrary shape. The measurement systems include 2D and 3D system setups, the choice of antenna, antenna positions and test objects.

4.1 System design

Figure 4-1 displays a possible implementation of a 3D HMI system (Wang et al., 2014a), which consisted of a single transmitter and an array of 15 receivers, a dielectric object (not showing) was placed on the window of an examination bed. All antennas were surrounding within the antenna array plane, which were connected to a 15-channel switch. The antenna array plane was placed under the examination bed in the far-field region of the array ($>6\lambda$) and it was designed to be moveable toward the target object in a vertical position. The dielectric object phantom was placed at $z = 0$ mm and the antenna array was placed under the object which was movable from $z = H_1$ mm to $z = H_n$ mm in equal M steps.

The two-port vector network analyzer (VNA) generates a single frequency microwave signal to the single transmitting antenna that transmits the electromagnetic (EM) wave into the object through the air where it is scattered in different directions. Each receiving antenna receives the backscattered electric field from the object. These measurements were repeated every time when the antenna array moved to a new position (change the measurement heights between the phantom and the antenna array plane). Microwave measurements that contain phase and magnitude of the reflection coefficient information were obtained using a VNA.

The complex visibility function was calculated using the measured data, and the 2D object intensity distribution was formed by applying an Inverse Fast Fourier Transform (IFFT) to the complex visibility data. A 2D projection image of a 3D dielectric object was then formed from the object intensity distribution when the antenna array plane was placed at the selected height. Then a 3D dielectric object image was

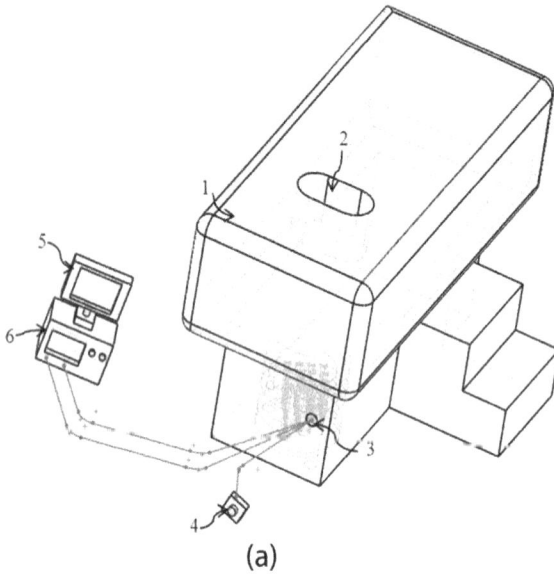

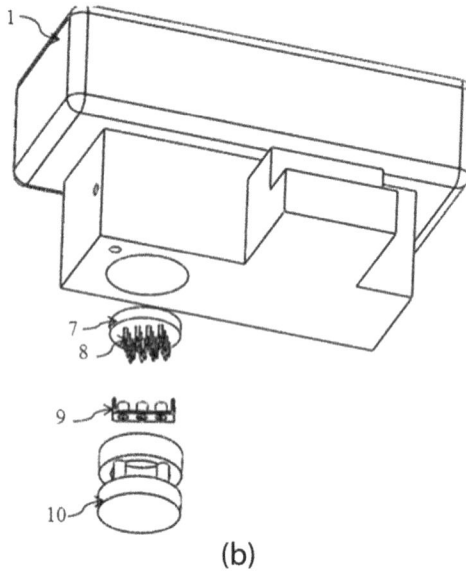

Figure 4-1 (a) 3D holographic microwave imaging system (b) bottom view of examination bed (1: examination bed, 2: examination window, 3: connection hole to antennas, 4: multi-position switch, 5: computer, 6: microwave generator, 7: antenna array plane, 8: antennas, 9: multi-position switch assembly, 10: antenna array holder) (Wang et al., 2014a).

reconstructed by using the 3D HMI image reconstruction algorithm with the antenna array plane placed at different heights.

4.2 Model and material

To evaluate the performance of the proposed technique, a dielectric object was used to verify the main characteristics of the system such as contrast, spatial resolution, size and positioning accuracy. The cube-shaped dielectric object consisted of an external cube made from an embedding medium and an inclusion. The external cube I made from emulsifying ointment that contained 30% emulsifying wax, 50% white soft paraffin and 20% liquid paraffin. The external cube II made of 90% emulsifying ointment and 10% water. Small grapes (7 mm to 15 mm in diameter) were inserted into the cube object to represent inclusion I. A small blueberry (9 mm in diameter) was inserted into the cube object to represent inclusion II. The dielectric object was covered by a thin plastic film to minimize moisture loss and to make the object easier to handle. The plastic film has a negligible effect on the scattered electromagnetic field in the considered frequency range. Air ($\varepsilon_r = 1$) was used as the medium filling the space between the dielectric object and antenna array.

4.3 Dielectric properties measurement

The actual dielectric properties of the external cube and inclusion were measured before 3D HMI data collection. Measurements with frequencies ranging from 10 GHz to 20 GHz were conducted using Agilent N5230A VNA and an Agilent 85070 single port dielectric probe. Reflection coefficients were converted to dielectric permittivity and loss tangent using Agilent 85070 dielectric measurement software. A dielectric kit open-ended coaxial probe was connected to the network analyzer for calibration.

Probe calibration was carried out using three calibration standards: air, short-circuit and finally deionized water at a temperature of 21°C. Following calibration, the probe was pressed against the sample ensuring no air gaps between sample and probe. The reflection coefficient was measured and used to determine the permittivity. Data was recorded at 101 frequency points between 10 GHz to 20 GHz. This measurement was repeated three times in order to get an average reading. The sample must be thick enough to appear effectively semi-infinite to the probe. After measuring each object, the probe was cleaned with tissue paper to prevent any oil that may accumulate on it during measurements. The

Table 4-1 Dielectric properties of materials at 12.6 GHz.

Material	Real part of permittivity	Imaginary part of permittivity	Size (mm)
External cube I (100% wax)	2.43	0.24	180 by 160 by 40; 100 by 100 by 30; 100 by 100 by 30
External cube (90% wax and 10% water)	3.16	0.53	100 by 100 by 40
Inclusion I (Grape)	21.23	19.3	Diameters: 4, 5, 7, 10, 15
Inclusion II (Blueberry)	27.73	7.98	Diameter: 9

measured electrical properties at 12.6 GHz ($\lambda = 23.8$ mm) of the external cube and inclusion are listed in Table 4-1.

4.4 Experimental system setup

Figure 4-2 shows the photograph of an initial 3D HMI data acquisition system. An array of 16 open-ended rectangular wave-guide antennas were surrounded with ECCOSORB AN79 (600 mm by 600 mm) electromagnetic absorbing material to reduce ambient reflections, and antennas were positioned as shown in Figure 4-3. Optimization of the antenna array configuration to produce high-resolution images will be presented in the next chapter. A small open-ended rectangular wave-guide antenna was selected as a transmitter and receiver in all experiments because of its low-cost and ease of manufacture. The antenna array was connected to an Agilent N5230A (10 GHz to 20 GHz) VNA. The target object was placed on the top of the polystyrene box bridge. The target object was located at a height above the antenna array plane that was varied between $z = 540$ mm (22.7λ) to $z = 550$ mm (23λ) in 11 equal steps by using two lab jacks. A height gauge was used to measure the target object movements of 1 mm increments and a spirit level was used to balance the polystyrene box bridge during movement.

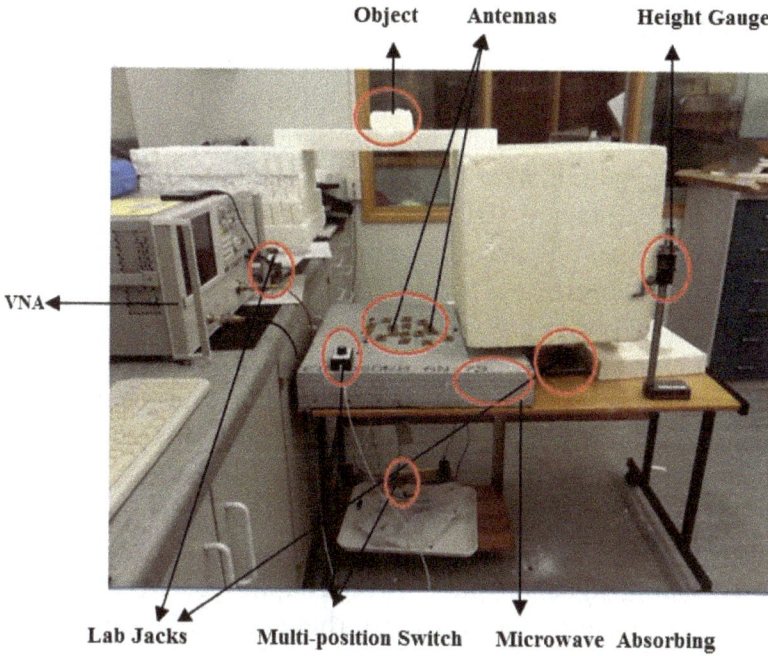

Figure 4-2   3D HMI system setup (Wang et al., 2014b).

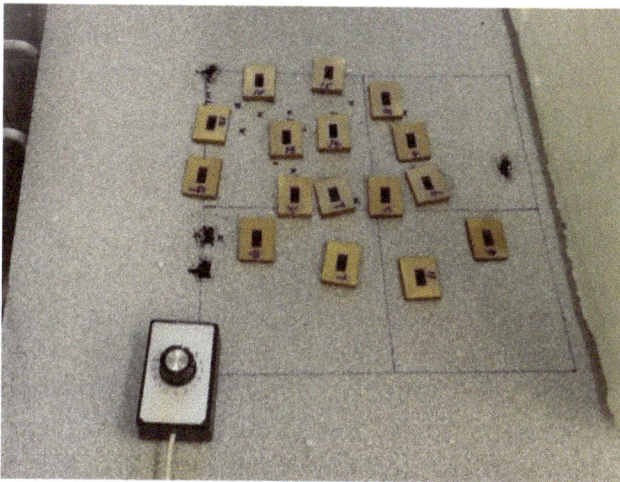

Figure 4-3   Photograph of antenna array configuration.

4.5   Data acquisition

Although only a single frequency was used for reconstructing the image, the wide frequency spectrum from 10 GHz to 20 GHz was collected so that the optimal frequency could be determined. Data was recorded at 3201 frequency points for choosing the optimum frequency between 10 GHz to 20 GHz and 101 measurements were averaged at each frequency. All 16 antennas were tested before data acquisition with one antenna as the transmitter and the others as the receivers. Background data (that is, with no object present) was collected at each receiver with the antenna array plane placed at $z = 540$ mm (22.7λ) before measuring the target object. This step was repeated three times and the data averaged. The dielectric object was illuminated by the transmitter and the real and imaginary parts of the backscattered field recorded at each receiver at the operating frequency of 12.6 GHz ($\lambda = 23.8$ mm). These data collection steps were repeated for every new vertical position of the antenna array.

The measured signals include direct coupling between the antennas and reflections from the target object, therefore calibration is necessary to remove coupling noise. In this study, the calibration signal was the average of background measurements, that is, with no test object present. This measured signal was subtracted from the actual response recorded for the target object at each receiving antenna. This step was repeated for every new vertical position of the antenna array. The antenna coupling signal was obtained both without the target object present in the measurement (background) and with the image. Images of all tested objects were reconstructed by using the developed imaging algorithms (referring to Chapter 3).

4.6   Imaging results

Figure 4-4 shows the dielectric object consisting of external cube I (100 mm by 100 mm by 30 mm) with inclusion I (10 mm in diameter), where the inclusion I is located at ($X = 50$ mm, $Y = 50$ mm, $Z = 10$ mm).

Figure 4-5 shows the reconstructed image (modulus part) of the object. The inclusion is clearly visible in the image at the correct location.

Figure 4-6 shows the dielectric object consisting of external cube I (180 mm by 160 mm by 40 mm) and two inclusions of type I (10 mm and 15 mm in diameter), where the inclusions are located at ($X_1 = 95$ mm, $Y_1 = 95$ mm, $Z_1 = 25$ mm) and ($X_2 = 138$ mm, $Y_2 = 40$ mm, $Z_2 = 25$ mm). The distance between two inclusions is approximately 69.8 mm (2.9λ).

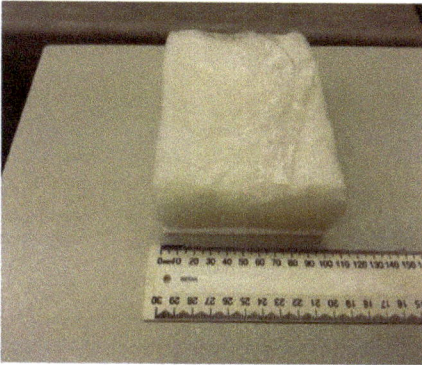
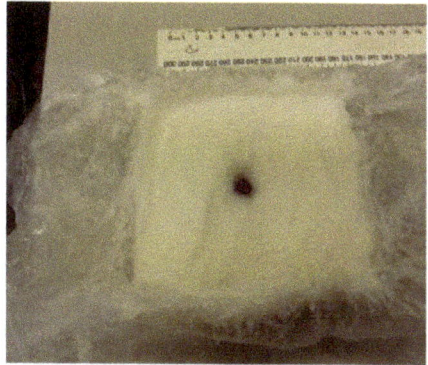

(a) (b)

Figure 4-4   Photograph of the target object, including one inclusion I (10 mm in diameter) (a) top view (b) inside view.

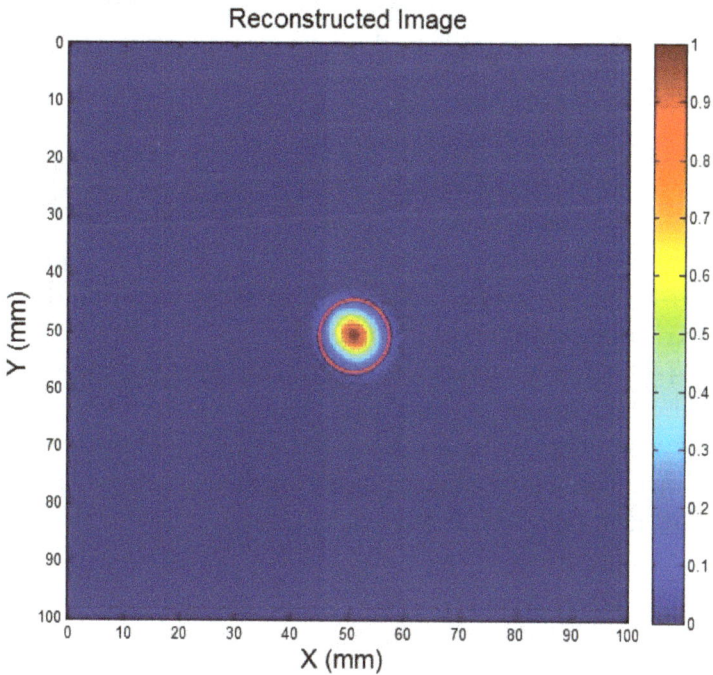

Figure 4-5   Image of dielectric object with one inclusion.

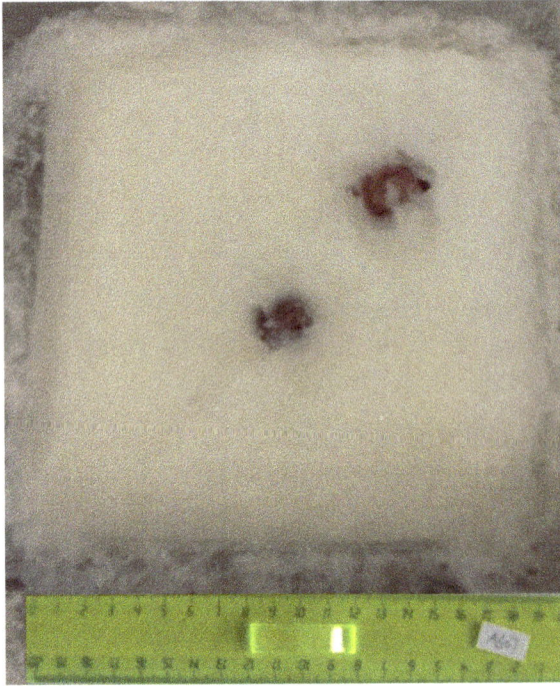

Figure 4-6   Photograph of the cube including two inclusions I.

Figure 4-7 displays the reconstructed image (modulus part) of the object. It clearly shows two inclusions in the reconstructed 3D image at the correct locations.

Figure 4-8 shows a single 2D slice of the reconstructed 3D image for the dielectric object shown in Figure 4-9.

Figure 4-10 shows a dielectric object consisting of external cube II (100 mm by 100 mm by 40 mm) and one inclusion of type II (9 mm in diameter) where the inclusion is located at (X = 50 mm, Y = 50 mm, Z = 35 mm). The whole object placed on the top of the antenna array at Z = 540 mm (22.7λ). Figure 4.11 shows a single 2D slice of the reconstructed 3D image.

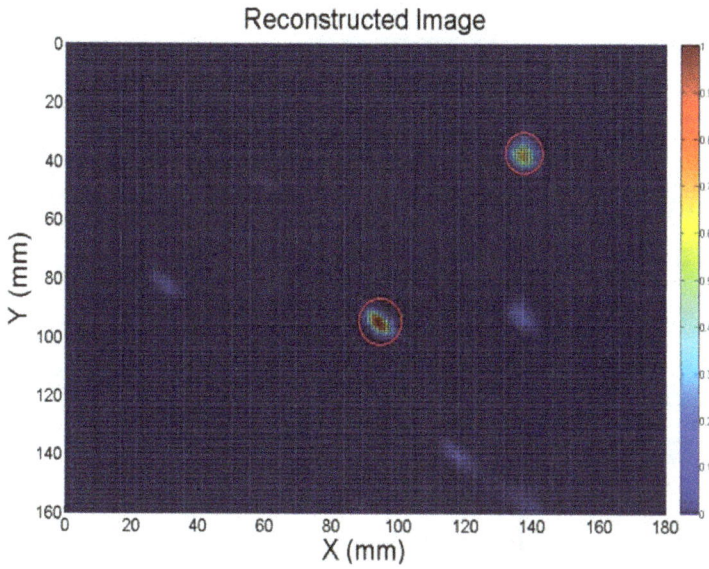

(a)

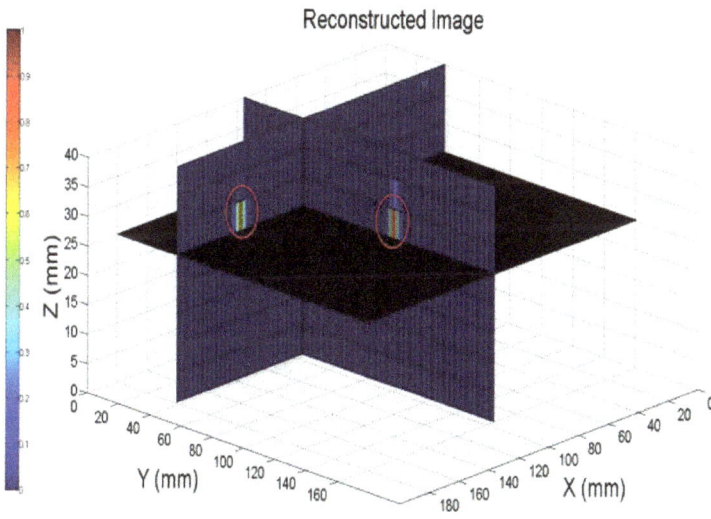

(b)

Figure 4-7   3D images with two inclusions I (a) top view (b) side views.

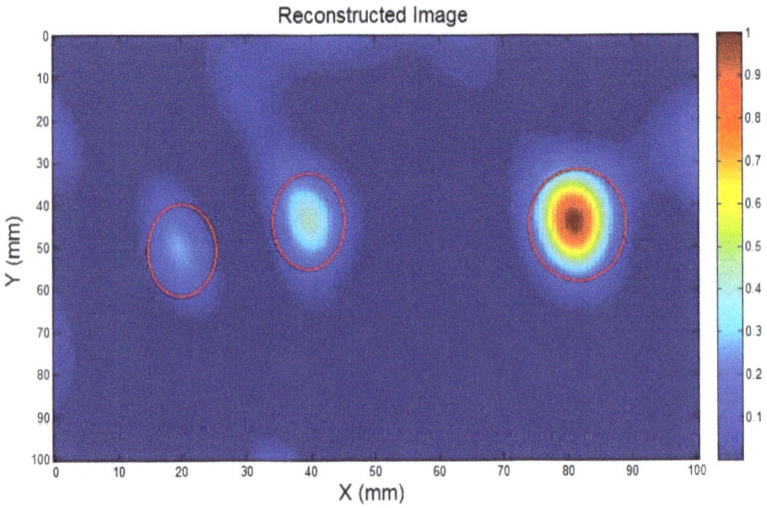

Figure 4-8   2D image showing three inclusions of type I.

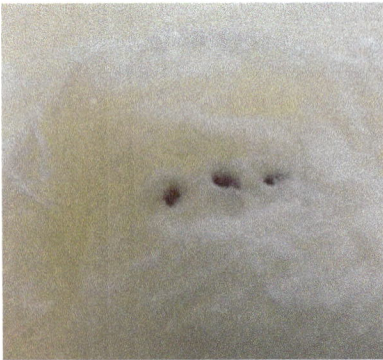

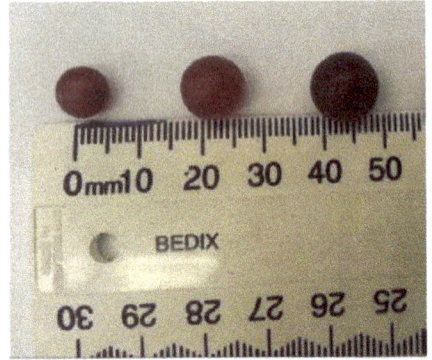

(a)   (b)

Figure 4-9   (a) Photograph of the dielectric object, including cube I and three inclusions of type I (b) size of inclusions
(4 mm, 5 mm, 7 mm in diameters).

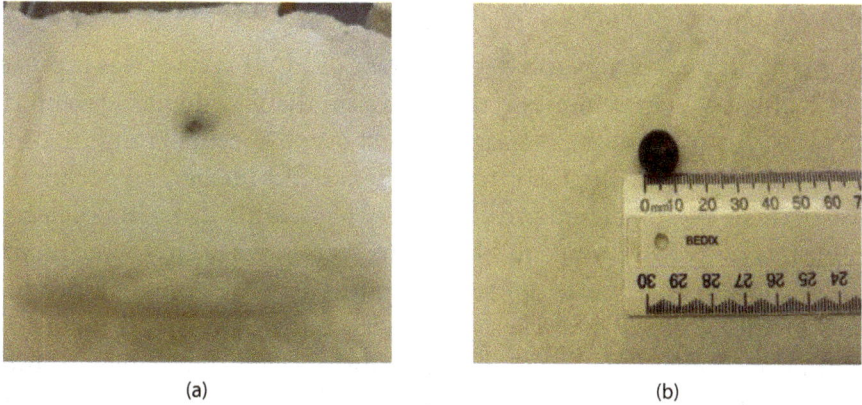

(a)   (b)

Figure 4-10   (a) Photograph of the dielectric object, including cube II and one inclusion of type II (b) size of inclusion (9 mm in diameter).

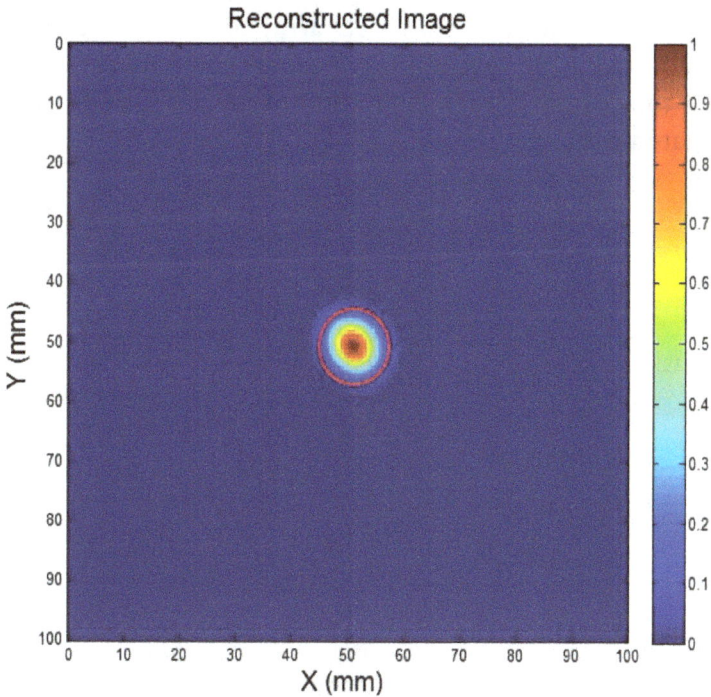

Figure 4-11   2D slice taken from 3D image showing single inclusion of type II.

4.7 Closure

The preliminary analysis and development of HMI system was reported in this chapter. The technique uses physical displacement between the antenna array plane and the imaged object over a specified range in order to obtain depth information from sequence 2D images. Experimental investigation of multimedia dielectric objects with different dielectric properties (contrast), sizes and locations were presented. Experimental results showed that the proposed technique has the ability to produce good quality images of dielectric objects and detect small inclusions within the object. The data collection time was approximately 10 minutes for 15 receivers at one selected height, while the CPU time required to produce a 2D image was approximately 0.5 second on an Intel Core (TM) i5 3.2 GHz with 8 GB RAM. The time required to measure 15 receivers at 10 different heights was approximately 100 minutes, while the CPU time required to produce a 3D image was approximately 1 minute on an Intel Core (TM) i5 3.2 GHz with 8 GB RAM. The image resolution depends on the antenna baseline difference, in other words, the antenna locations on a 2D array plane. A matching medium was not required in this preliminary experiment, only air, which greatly simplified the practical implementation of such a system and reduced the associated cost.

5. Antenna and antenna arrays

Antenna array configuration plays an important role in HMI measurement system. This chapter demonstrates optimization of various antenna array configurations to generate a high-resolution image of dielectric objects by using the proposed technique. Three configurations include spiral, random and regularly spaced array are presented in this chapter, both simulation and experimental results are obtained and compared to fully demonstrate the effectiveness of antenna arrays to the HMI technique.

5.1 Introduction

The performance of producing high-resolution microwave images at lower costs have been investigated by many researchers (Hagness et al., 1998; Fear et al., 2002), which includes antenna design, optimization of antenna array configuration (also named as array geometry) and investigation of image algorithms. Planar (Bond et al., 2003) and circular (Fear et al., 2013) antenna array configurations are the two most common types of antenna arrays in microwave biological imaging. Both of them are regularly spaced array configurations. Circular array configuration is more suitable for the clinical environment and the use of more antennas would provide higher resolution images and are more sensitive to small tumors. To generate a high-resolution microwave image, the existing antenna arrays require a large number of antennas which can be as large as several hundreds. The performance of an antenna array (for whatever application it is being used) increases with the number of antennas in the array. The limitations include the increased cost, size, and complexity. In general, the radiation pattern of an antenna array depends on the weighting method and the geometry of the array. However, the array configurations especially in biomedical imaging applications have received relatively little attention even though it strongly influences the radiation pattern.

5.2 Antenna and antenna array configurations

5.2.1 Antenna design

The flanged open-ended rectangular waveguide antenna (ORWA) was selected as transmitter and receivers due to the following benefits:

+ It is compact enough to be located on to a scanning arrangement

- It is cost effective and widely available
- The antenna is easy to move and relocated on the array plane to study the performance of antenna array
- The small size also allowed for the positioning of many antennas close to the imaging domain

Figure 5-1(a) shows a schematic of the designed ORWA. The excitation port P was placed at 9 mm from the end of the waveguide and the dimensions are listed in Table 5-1. The WR62 waveguide that has a cut-off frequency of 9.5 GHz was used to design the ORWA as shown in Figure 5-1(b) (Wang et al., 2015). A small Male SMA connector was inserted through the sidewall of the waveguide and was placed at 9 mm from the bottom of the antenna (termination) as the excitation port. This enabled the waveguide to be connected with an RG coaxial cable for measurement and analysis.

5.2.2   Antenna array configurations

Figure 5-2 displays the geometry relevant to the HMI imaging, where x, y and z represent antenna locations in the array plane. If a point $P(x,y,z)$ is assumed in the target dielectric object, under far-field conditions, the 2D image of projected scattering intensity within the dielectric object $\tilde{I}(l,m)$ is:

$$\tilde{I}(l,m) = \iint G(u,v)e^{j2\pi(ul+vm)}dudv \qquad (5\text{-}1)$$

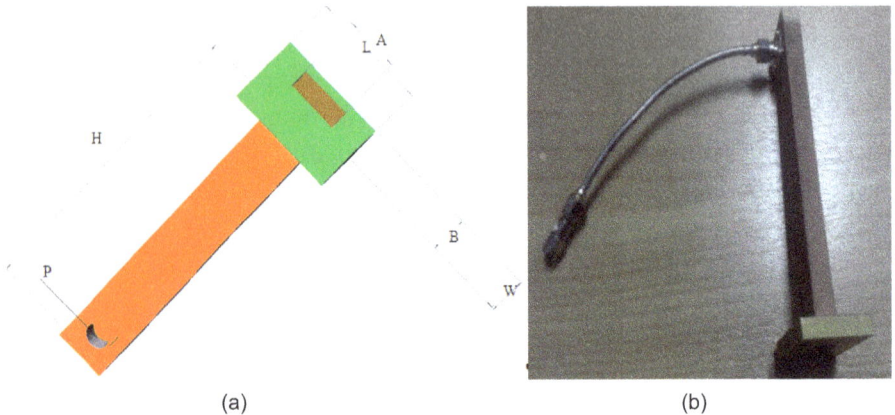

(a)   (b)

Figure 5-1   (a) Configuration of flanged ORWA (b) photography of the flanged ORWA with connection cable.

Table 5-1 Dimensions of flanged ORWA (Wang et al., 2015).

Parameter	Dimension (mm)
Width of waveguide (A)	15.8
Length of waveguide (B)	7.9
Height of waveguide (H)	120
Thickness of the waveguide walls	1
Length of flange (L)	38
Width of flange (W)	2
Thickness of the flange (T)	6
Length of excitation port from the end of waveguide (P)	9

Where (l,m) was defined as $(\sin\theta \cos\phi, \sin\theta \sin\phi)$, refers to the polar coordinates as shown in Figure 5-2. $G(u,v)$ is the complex visibility data which was detailed in Chapter 3.

In HMI system, all antennas were assumed to be located on a 2D plane. The U-V coverage was developed for optimization of the antenna

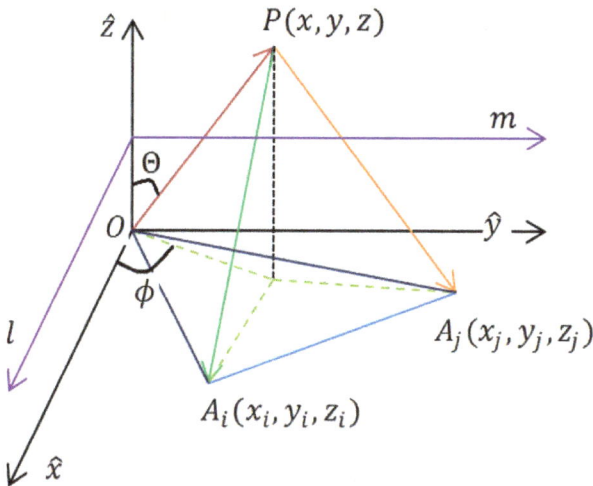

Figure 5-2 Geometry of HMI measurement by one pair of antenna.

array configuration and object image. For any given pair of antennas $A_i(x_i,y_i,z_i)$ and $A_j(x_j,y_j,z_j)$, U-V coverage can be defined as:

$$(u_{ij}, v_{ij}) = (x_j - x_i, y_j - y_i)/\lambda \qquad (5\text{-}2)$$

Where λ is the wavelength in free space.

Baseline B is equal to the difference between the antenna positions over the XY plane normalized to the wavelength in free space, can be calculated by:

$$B_{ij} = \sqrt{(u_{ij})^2 + (v_{ij})^2} \qquad (5\text{-}3)$$

Equation (5-1) performs the 2D dielectric object image. The development of the 2D HMI imaging algorithm is detailed in Chapter 3.

In order to design an antenna array plane that is more suitable for medical imaging applications using the HMI technique with lower cost and less operation time, the following factors need to be considered:

- The antenna array plane should contain as few antennas as possible
- The antenna array should be able to provide dense sampling of the aperture (U-V coverage) over a wide range of projected baseline values
- The antenna array should be able to offer the best possibility of detecting lesions anywhere within the target dielectric object

A computer simulation model was developed to investigate antenna array configurations effect on image quality by using HMI applications. The authors investigated hundreds of antenna arrays, this chapter only presents and compares the selected spiral array, random array and regularly spaced array.

Antenna locations on a logical spiral array flat plane (2D) can be obtained by:

$$x = \frac{L(t\cos(t) + \min\|t\cos(t)\|)}{\max\|t\cos(t)\| + \min\|t\cos(t)\|}$$

$$\qquad (5\text{-}4)$$

$$y = \frac{W(t\sin(t) + \min\|t\sin(t)\|)}{\max\|t\sin(t)\| + \min\|t\sin(t)\|}$$

Where $t = linespace(a\pi,\pi/b,N)$, a = Anticlockwise rotation angle, b = Clockwise rotation angle, N = Antenna number, L = Antenna array plane length, W = Antenna plane width.

Antenna locations on a random flat array plane can be calculated by using MATLAB random function:

$$(x,y) = rand(N,2) \times L \qquad (5\text{-}5)$$

Where N = Antenna number, L = Antenna array plane length.

5.3 Simulation

5.3.1 Antenna array configurations

A mathematical computer simulation model was developed using MATLAB to performance images using various antenna array configurations. This program quickly calculates and displays the U-V coverage of antenna arrays by combination of Equations (5-2), (5-4) and (5-5). All antennas are located on a flat plane (300 mm by 300 mm). Three 16-element antenna array planes are shown in Figure 5-3, with one acting as transmitting antenna and the remaining sensors acting as receiving antennas. The antenna locations on different array configurations are listed in Table 5-2.

5.3.2 Target dielectric object

Figure 5-4 shows a 2D view of the hemispherical shaped dielectric model (radius of 70 mm) with two spherical inclusions located at the same layer within the object. This dielectric object is used to simulate a multi-media dielectric model that contains 2 mm thick substructure1 ($\varepsilon_r = 9.3$, $\sigma = 4$ S/m), substructure2 ($\varepsilon_r = 9$, $\sigma = 0.4$ S/m) and two inclusions ($\varepsilon_r = 9.5$, $\sigma = 7$ S/m) of 5 mm in diameter. The space between the object and antenna array was assumed to be filled with air ($\varepsilon_r = 1$, $\sigma = 0$ S/m). The model was placed at $z = 0$ mm and all antenna array configurations were placed at $z = -450$ mm. Color bar describes the complex relative permittivity of the dielectric object.

5.3.3 Signal and imaging processing

During operation, one port of a microwave generator excites the single transmitter at one frequency of 12.6 GHz (Wang et al., 2014b). The magnitude and phase of the backscattered electric field from the target object was measured at each receiver element in the array plane, which

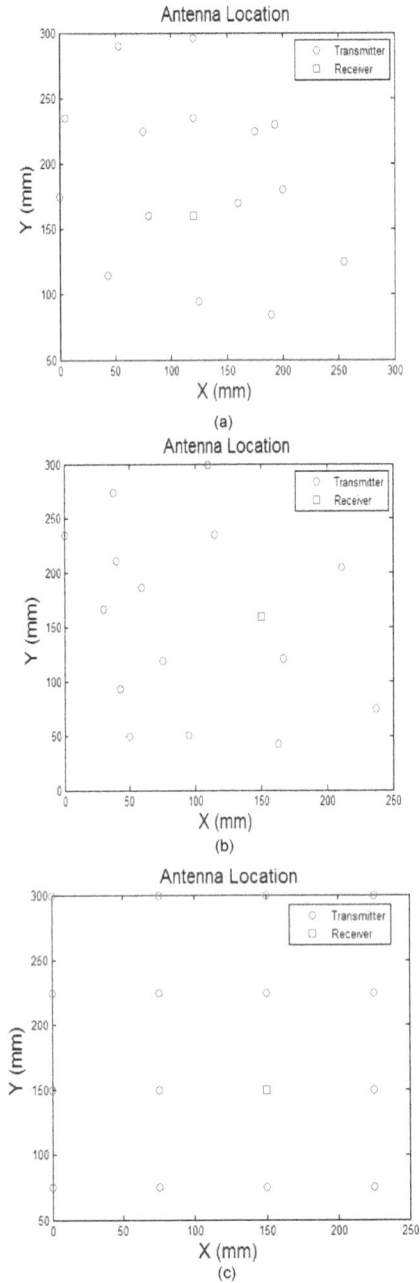

Figure 5-3 (a) Spiral antenna array configuration (b) random antenna array configuration (c) regular spaced antenna array configuration.

Table 5-2 Antenna location on different array planes.

	Spiral antenna array				Random antenna array				Regular spaced			
Rx	X (mm)	Y (mm)	Scale value of X to array plane length	Scale value of Y to array plane width	X (mm)	Y (mm)	Scale value of X to array plane length	Scale value of Y to array plane width	X (mm)	Y (mm)	Scale value of X to array plane length	Scale value of Y to array plane width
1	80	160	0.27	0.53	43	94	0.14	0.31	75	150	0.25	0.50
2	200	180	0.67	0.60	50	50	0.17	0.17	0	75	0.00	0.25
3	160	170	0.53	0.57	237	75	0.79	0.25	225	150	0.75	0.50
4	190	85	0.63	0.28	167	121	0.56	0.40	150	75	0.50	0.25
5	255	125	0.85	0.42	95	51	0.32	0.17	75	75	0.25	0.25
6	125	95	0.42	0.32	163	43	0.54	0.14	225	75	0.75	0.25
7	175	225	0.58	0.75	115	235	0.38	0.78	150	225	0.50	0.75
8	0	175	0	0.58	30	167	0.10	0.56	0	225	0	0.75
9	53	290	0.18	0.97	59	187	0.20	0.62	75	300	0.25	1.00

(Continued)

Table 5-2 Antenna location on different array planes. (*Continued*)

Rx	Spiral antenna array				Random antenna array				Regular spaced			
	X (mm)	Y (mm)	Scale value of X to array plane length	Scale value of Y to array plane width	X (mm)	Y (mm)	Scale value of X to array plane length	Scale value of Y to array plane width	X (mm)	Y (mm)	Scale value of X to array plane length	Scale value of Y to array plane width
10	120	296	0.40	0.99	0	235	0.00	0.78	150	300	0.50	1.00
11	5	235	0.02	0.78	38	274	0.13	0.91	0	300	0.00	1.00
12	75	225	0.25	0.75	40	212	0.13	0.71	75	225	0.25	0.75
13	120	235	0.40	0.78	211	205	0.70	0.68	225	225	0.75	0.75
14	193	230	0.64	0.77	110	300	0.37	1.00	225	300	0.75	1.00
15	43	115	0.14	0.38	75	119	0.25	0.40	0	150	0	0.50
Tx	120	160	0.4	0.53	150	160	0.5	0.53	150	150	0.5	0.5

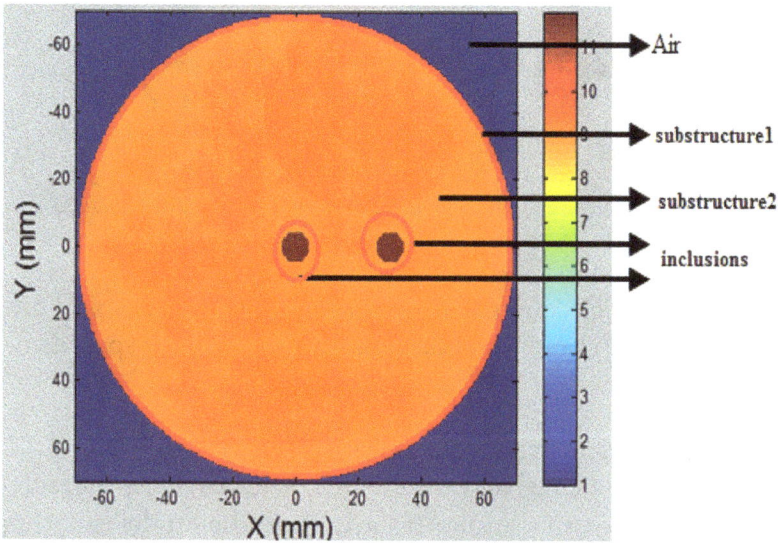

Figure 5-4   Original model under test.

was connected to the second port of the microwave generator via a 16-channel switch. These measurements were repeated for every new vertical position of the antenna array plane. The complex valued data measured at each receiving antenna can be used to calculate the complex visibility data for each possible pair of antennas. The complex visibility data then used to form a 2D image using an inverse Fourier transform. A computer with MATLAB software was used to analyse the reflected singles and perform images of the object under test by using the developed HMI imaging algorithms.

5.3.4   Simulation results

Figure 5-5 shows the reconstructed 2D images using the spiral, random and regularly spaced array configurations, respectively. Figure 5-6 compares the reconstructed images using a 16-element random antenna array. The antenna array plane was varied between $z = -50$ mm and $z = -600$ mm in 12 equal steps and the dielectric object was placed at $z = 0$ mm. Color bars in Figure 5-5 indicate the backscattered field from the dielectric object on a linear scale, normalized to the maximum in the 2D images space.

Table 5-3 compares the simulation results (inclusion detection quantitative) that were obtained by using three different array configurations. Table 5-4 summaries the simulation results of the same dielectric object

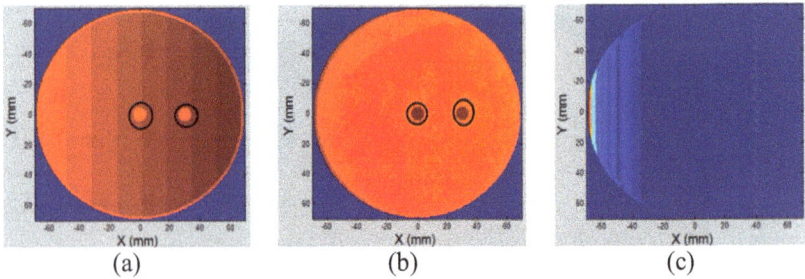

Figure 5-5 Reconstructed 2D images using: (a) spiral antenna array (b) random antenna array (c) regularly spaced antenna array.

by using a 16-element random antenna array configuration but the dielectric object was placed at a different height. The best measurement distance range between the antenna array and the model is 450 mm to 550 mm (see Figure 5-6). Measurement height out of the best range can cause artefacts and these make it difficult to identify lesions on the reconstructed images.

5.4   Experimental

5.4.1   Model and materials

A dielectric object was used to test the proposed antenna array configurations. The cube-shaped dielectric object consisted of an external cube made from an embedding medium and an inclusion. The external cube was made from emulsifying ointment that contained 30% emulsifying wax, 50% white soft paraffin and 20% liquid paraffin. Small grapes were inserted into the cube object to represent inclusion. The dielectric object was covered by a thin plastic film to minimize moisture loss and to make the object easier to handle. The plastic film has a negligible effect on the scattered electromagnetic field in the considered frequency range. Air ($\varepsilon_r = 1$) was used as the medium filling the space between the dielectric object and antenna array.

5.4.2   Dielectric properties measurement

The actual dielectric properties of the external cube and inclusion were measured. Measurements with frequencies ranging from 10 GHz to 20 GHz were conducted using Agilent N5230A VNA and an Agilent 85070 single port dielectric probe. Reflection coefficients were converted to dielectric permittivity and loss tangent using Agilent 85070 dielectric

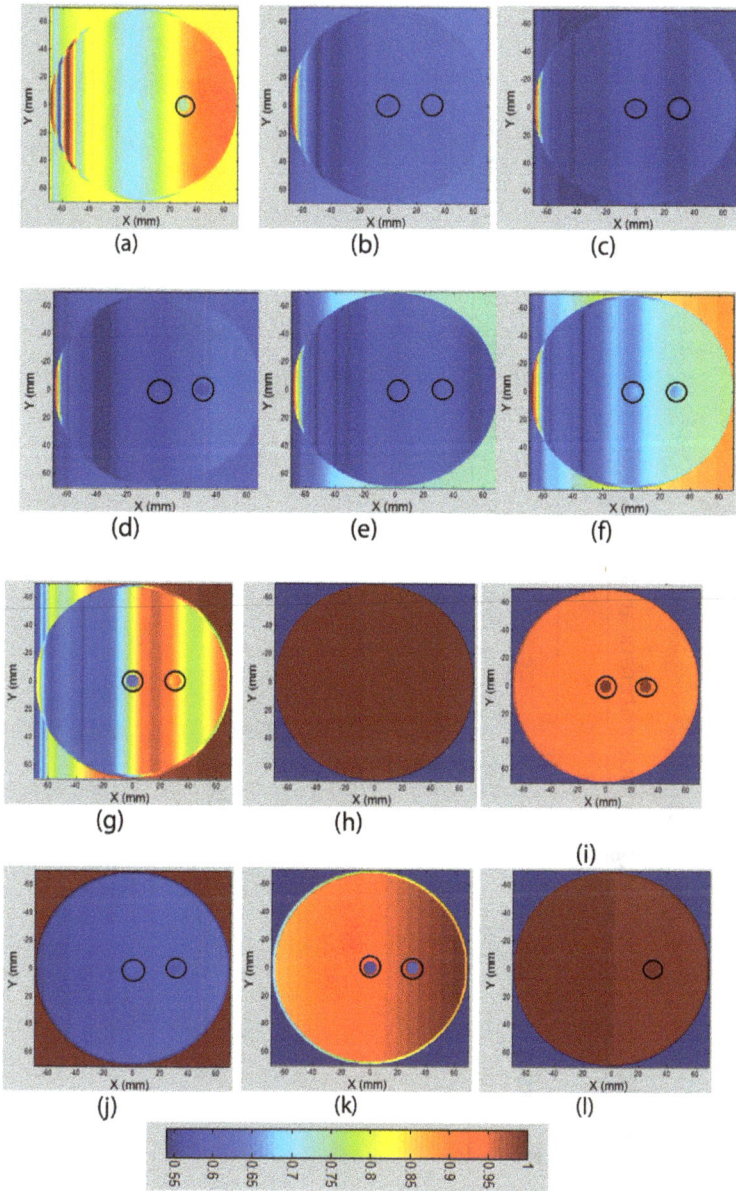

Figure 5-6 2D reconstructed object images with random antenna array was placed at (a) $z = -50$ mm (b) $z = -100$ mm (c) $z = -150$ mm (d) $z = -200$ mm (e) $z = -250$ mm (f) $z = -300$ mm (g) $z = -350$ mm (h) $z = -400$ mm (i) $z = -450$ mm (j) $z = -500$ mm (k) $z = -550$ mm (l) $z = -600$ mm.

Table 5-3 Simulation results using various antenna array configurations.

Array	Transmitter no.	Receiver no.	Density	Size (mm)	Inclusions No.	Locations	Detection	Artifacts
Spiral	1	15	0.289	5	2	$x_1 = 0,$ $y_1 = 0,$ $z_1 = 20,$ $x_2 = 30,$ $y_2 = 0,$ $z_2 = 20$	2	No
Random			0.269				2	No
Regularly spaced			0.0255				0	Yes

Table 5-4 Simulation results using random array configuration at different measurement heights.

Height (mm)	Transmitter no.	Receiver no.	Density	Size (mm)	Inclusions Locations	Detection	Artifacts
50	1	15	0.269	5		1	Yes
100						2	Yes
150						2	Yes
200						1	Yes
250					$x_1 = 0,$ $y_1 = 0,$ $z_1 = 20,$ $x_2 = 30,$ $y_2 = 0,$ $z_2 = 20$	2	Yes
300						2	Yes
350						2	Yes
400						0	Yes
450						2	No
500						2	No
550						2	No
600						1	No

Table 5-5 Dielectric properties of materials at 12.6 GHz.

Material	Real part of permittivity	Imaginary part of permittivity	Size (mm)
External cube (100% wax)	2.43	0.24	100 by 100 by 30
Inclusion (Grape)	21.23	19.3	Diameters: 10

measurement software. A dielectric kit open-ended coaxial probe was connected to the network analyser for calibration. Probe calibration was carried out using three calibration standards: air, short-circuit and finally deionized water at a temperature of 21°C. Following calibration, the probe was pressed against the sample ensuring no air gaps between sample and probe. The reflection coefficient was measured and used to determine the permittivity. Data was recorded at 101 frequency points between 10 GHz to 20 GHz. This measurement was repeated three times in order to get an average reading. The sample must be thick enough to appear effectively semi-infinite to the probe. After measuring each object, the probe was cleaned with tissue paper to prevent any oil that may accumulate on it during measurements. The measured dielectric properties at 12.6 GHz of the external cube and inclusion are listed in Table 5-5.

5.4.3   Experimental system setup

An experimental verification of the antenna arrays using the HMI technique was performed. Figure 4-2 shows an experimental setup of HMI data acquisition system (Wang et al., 2014b). Figure 5-7 displays the experimental setups of three antenna array configurations. The calibration and data acquisition processing were demonstrated in Chapter 4.

5.5   Imaging results and discuss

5.5.1   Reconstruction results

Figure 5-8 shows the dielectric object (100 mm by 100 mm by 30 mm) including an external cube I and two inclusions of type I (10 mm in diameter), where the inclusions are located at (X_1 = 50 mm, Y_1 = 50 mm, Z_1 = 20 mm) and (X_2 = 70 mm, Y_2 = 80 mm, Z_2 = 20 mm).

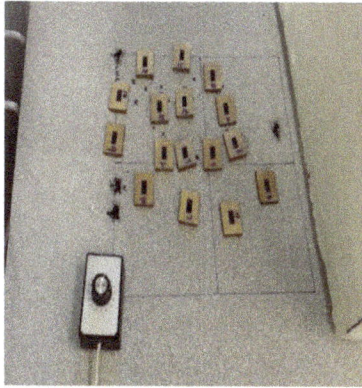

(a)

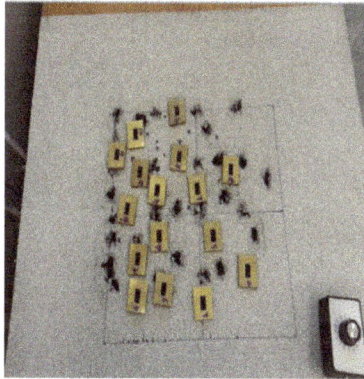

(b)

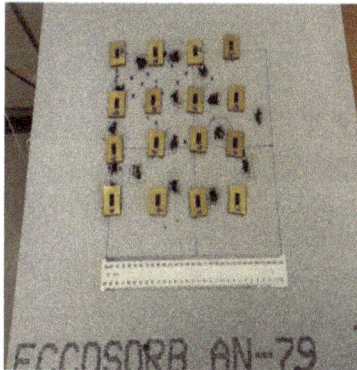

(c)

Figure 5-7 Experimental setup of antenna array planes (a) spiral array (b) random array (c) regularly spaced.

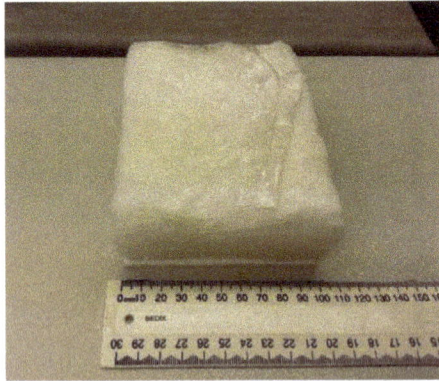

(a)

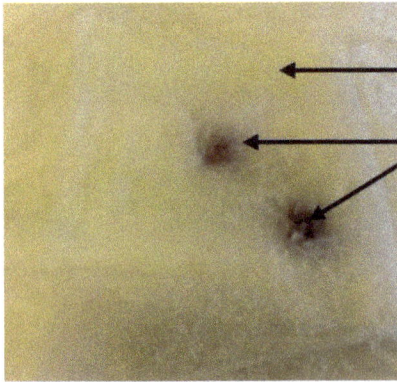

External cube

Dielectric
inclusions

(b)

Figure 5-8 Photograph of the cube including two inclusions (a) top view (b) inside view.

The 2D reconstructed images (modulus part) of a dielectric object with different antenna array configurations are shown in Figure 5-9. Results indicate that two inclusions are detected clearly within the reconstructed image when using spiral and random antenna arrays. As can be seen that inclusions are not represented in the reconstruction image when using regularly spaced antenna array. Color bars plot signal intensity on a linear scale that is normalized to the maximum in the 2D image space. Values below 0.1 are rendered as blue.

5.5.2   Discussion

The three selected antenna arrays were compared as shown in Table 5-6. A quantitative analysis provides useful insight into the imaging

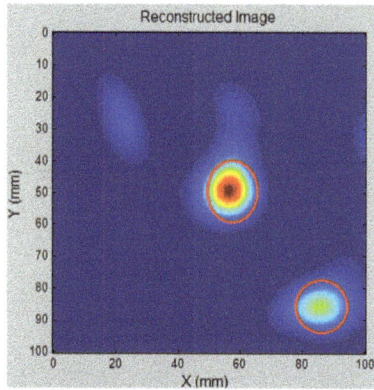

(a)

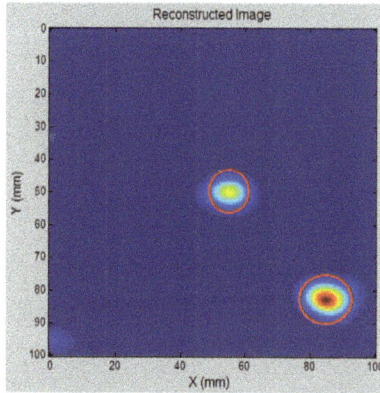

(b)

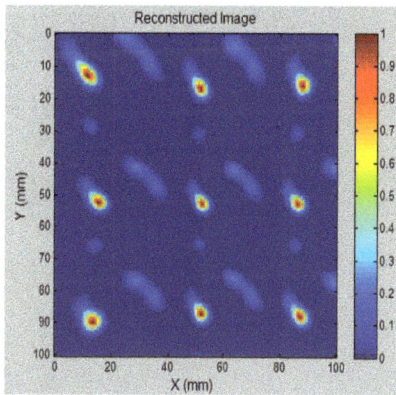

(c)

Figure 5-9   Reconstructed images of two inclusions using: (a) spiral antenna array (b) random antenna array (c) regularly spaced antenna array.

Table 5-6 Comparison of various antenna arrays.

Arrays	Spiral	Random	Regularly spaced
U-V coverage			
Density	0.1817	0.1870	0.0176
Minimum baseline	0.7846	1.3188	3.1500
Average baseline	3.1258	3.4137	3.9387
Unique baseline number	103	106	10
Spatial resolution	0.1234, 0.1128	0.1128, 0.0926	0.1058, 0.1058

performance of antenna array. U-V density was defined as the maximum U-V coverage value in the antenna array divided by the array plane size (mm^2). There is a significant difference of density, maximum, minimum, average and unique baseline between spiral, random and regularly spaced antenna arrays. Spiral and random arrays provide significantly more dense sampling on the aperture plane over a wide range of the baseline than regularly spaced array (0.1817 vs. 0.0176). The image resolution depends on density and unique baseline (different baseline) numbers in the antenna array, the sensitivity is determined by the minimum and average baseline in the antenna array. Results show that lesions were successfully detected using the spiral and random array configurations but cannot be easily identified by visualization using the regularly spaced array configuration. It seems that image resolution is determined by the U-V density and unique baseline number in the antenna array plane. Higher value of U-V density with more unique baseline number produces a better quality microwave image. The experimental results illustrate a good agreement with simulation results. Results show that it is possible to produce a good quality dielectric object image using 16-element spiral and random arrays.

Compared to the 31-element and 64-element regular antenna arrays (Klemm et al., 2010), the proposed spiral and random arrays have advantages in reducing the system cost and the data acquisition time. Such antenna systems have many benefits, which include low cost, short scanning time, steer ability, compact, and simplicity of manufacturing process. The potential applications of the proposed logical spiral and random antenna array configurations would be medical imaging, such as breast imaging and head imaging. The main drawback of the proposed arrays includes: all obtained images using HMI technique that developed based on U-V coverage which are similar to the synthetic aperture radar technology in radio astronomy technology. Such antenna arrays may not be suitable for other microwave imaging approaches.

5.6 Closure

Various antenna array configurations were reported in this chapter. The experimental results achieved a good agreement with simulation results and further confirmed the promise of microwave screening for breast lesion. Both simulation and experimental results demonstrated that using the same element antenna arrays, the spiral and random antenna arrays deliver clearer and more accurate images than the regularly spaced configuration. Random antenna array also provides the highest value of U-V density and offers the best possibility of detecting lesions within the breast phantom. Compared to the current widely used regularly spaced array in microwave imaging applications, the proposed antenna arrays have some advantages, which include low cost, short scanning time, compact, easy to manufacturing, and easy to setup.

6. Potential Application I-Breast cancer detection

This chapter presents the feasibility and potential performance characteristics of the proposed technique for medical imaging applications, with a particular focus on breast cancer detection. Several computer models were developed using MATLAB to validate the theory.

6.1 Introduction

As demonstrated in Chapter 2, breast imaging is one of the most widely investigated applications of microwave imaging, which aims to detect breast cancer or tumor by using the microwave imaging approaches due to the relatively high contrast of the breast tumor compared to the prominent fat tissue in a breast.

6.2 Theory

Referring to Figure 6-1, a point $P(x,y,z)$ was assumed within a dielectric object, under far-field condition, the intensity distribution of the object $I(s)$ at position s:

$$I(s) = \begin{cases} \left[\left(\dfrac{k_b^2}{2}\right)^3 (\varepsilon(s) - \varepsilon_b)^2 E_T(s) \cdot E_T^*(s), \text{ for a 2D object} \\ \left(\dfrac{k_0^2}{4\pi}\right)^3 (\varepsilon(ss) - \varepsilon_b)^2 E_T(s) \cdot E_T^*(s), \text{ for a 3D object} \end{cases} \tag{6-1}$$

Where k_0 is the wave number in free space, k_b is the wave number in the host medium, $\varepsilon(s)$ is the complex relative permittivity distribution of the object, ε_b is the complex relative permittivity of the host medium and $E_T(s)$ is the total electric field (incident plus scattered) at a point inside the object with position vector s.

The baseline vector $\mathbf{D}$ of any two receivers can be written in Cartesian components as below:

$$\begin{aligned} u &= (x_j - x_i)/\lambda_b \\ v &= (y_j - y_i)/\lambda_b \\ w &= (z_j - z_i)/\lambda_b \end{aligned} \tag{6-2}$$

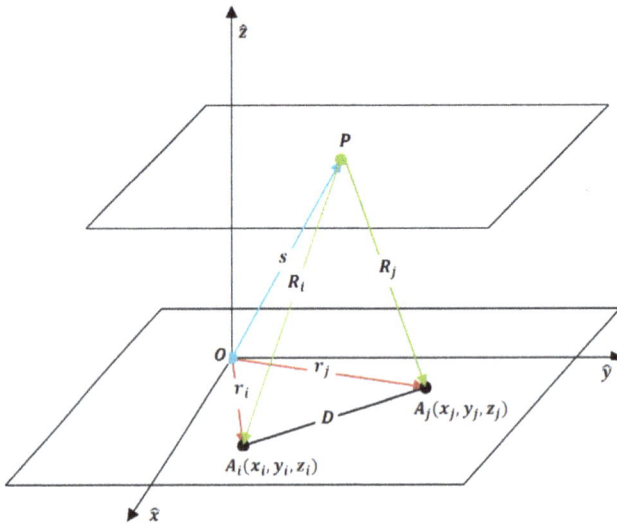

Figure 6-1 Geometry of HMI measurements by a pair of antennas.

The 2D intensity function of the object under test can be obtained:

$$\tilde{I}(l,m) = \iint G(u,v,w=0)e^{j2\pi(ul+vm)}dldm \qquad (6\text{-}3)$$

Equation (6-3) shows that a 2D image can be determined by Fourier inversion and it is a projection of the 3D intensity function onto a 2D plane in (l,m) space.

The 3D intensity function of the object at a selected height:

$$I(H = z_n, l, m) = d\tilde{I}(l,m) \cdot (1 - l^2 - m^2)/dz \qquad (6\text{-}4)$$

The derivative in Equation (6-4) can be approximated by the following forward difference expression:

$$\frac{d\tilde{I}}{dz} = \frac{\tilde{I}_{Z_n} - \tilde{I}_{Z_{n-1}}}{Z_n - Z_{n-1}} \qquad (6\text{-}5)$$

6.3 Simulation setups

6.3.1 System configuration

A computer model was developed to validate the HMI technique. One possible implementation of HMI system as presented in Figure 5-1. The examination bed contains a window that is made of material with

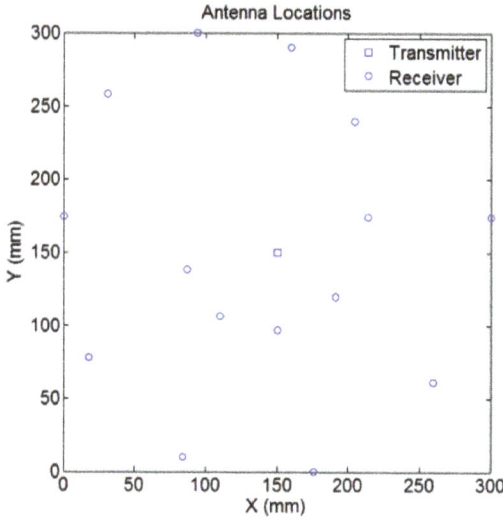

Figure 6-2 Antenna array configuration.

lossless dielectric material, and the object under test was placed in the window. A 16-element antenna array plane (see Figure 6-2) was placed and moved from $z = -460$ mm (19.3λ) to $z = -440$ mm (18.5λ) in 20 equal steps (0.4λ). The target object was located at $z = 0$ mm and was assumed to be fully contained in a rectangle imaging domain with length 150 mm (6.3λ). The space between the antenna array plane and the examination widow was filled with lossless dielectric material (same as examination window material).

6.3.2 Antenna

A small open-ended rectangular waveguide was assumed as both transmitter and receivers. The radiated far-field, E_{inc}, from such antenna is well-represented as:

$$E_{inc}(R,\theta,\varnothing) = \left(-\frac{jk_b}{2\pi^2}\right) E_0 \left(\frac{e^{-jk_b R_0}}{R_0}\right) ABh(\theta,\varnothing)P(\theta,\varnothing) \quad (6-6)$$

It is well-known that the backscattered field can be represented as an integral over the volume of the scatterer involving the induced polarization currents that arise from the complex permittivity contrast within the free space. The scattered field at any receiver can be found by applying the Stratton & Chu formulation (Silver, 1984):

$$E_{scat} = \frac{k_0^2}{4\pi} \int_V (\varepsilon(s) - \varepsilon_b)$$ (6-7)

$$\{aE_{tot}(s) + (bE_{tot}(s) \cdot \widehat{R})\widehat{R}\} \frac{e^{-jk_bR}}{R} dV$$

Where
$a = 1 - j/k_bR - 1/(k_bR)^2, b = -1 + 3j/k_bR + 3/(k_bR)^2$

When $k_bR \gg 1$, the above factors can be approximated by $a \approx 1$ and $b \approx 1$. For the purposes of demonstrating the HMI technique, it was computationally advantageous to consider a small permittivity contrast between the target and host medium thus $(\varepsilon(s) - \varepsilon_b)$ was assumed to be small. In this case, the backscattered field can be readily determined using the Born Approximation, which allows the total electric field, E_{tot}, to be approximated by the incident field, so that:

$$E_{scat}(r) = \left(\frac{k_0^2}{4\pi}\right) \int_V (\varepsilon(s) - \varepsilon_b)$$ (6-8)

$$\{E_{inc}(s) + (E_{inc}(s) \cdot \widehat{R})\widehat{R}\} \frac{e^{-jk_bR}}{R} dV$$

Assume $E_{inc}(s) \cdot \widehat{R} \approx 0$ referring to far-field condition, then the back-scattered field can be obtained:

$$E_{scat}(r) = \left(\frac{k_0^2}{4\pi}\right) \int_V (\varepsilon(s) - \varepsilon_b) E_{inc}(s) \frac{e^{-jk_bR}}{R} dV$$ (6-9)

6.3.3 Breast model

A 3D computer model was developed using MATLAB software by combining Equation (3-1) and Equation (6-9) to compute the complex visibility function. 3D images of the object under test governed by Equation (6-4) and Equation (6-5). To create 3D images using the 3D HMI technique, several dielectric objects including single and multiple small inclusions were considered. Table 6-1 summarizes the material, shape, size, and dielectric properties of models under test.

Table 6-1 Models under test.

Model	No.	Material	Shape	Thickness (mm)	Location (mm)			Dielectric properties		Scale value of dielectric properties	
					x	y	z	ε_r	σ(s/m)	ε_r	σ(s/m)
I	A_1	Medium	Cube	150	0	0	0	36	0	36	0
	A_2	Skin	Spherical	60	75	75	75	36	4	36	4
II	B_1	Medium	Cube	100	0	0	0	9	0	0.18	0
	B_2	Skin	Spherical	5	0	0	50	36	4	0.72	0.4
	B_3	Fat	Spherical	45	0	0	50	9	0.4	0.18	0.04
	B_4	Gland	Spherical	10	0	0	50	13	0.45	0.26	0.045
	B_5	Lesion	Spherical	4	0	0	50	50	0.4	1	0.04
III	C_1	Medium	Cube	100	0	0	0	9	0	0.18	0
	C_2	Skin	Spherical	5	0	0	50	36	4	0.72	0.4
	C_3	Fat	Spherical	45	0	0	50	9	0.4	0.18	0.04
	C_4	Lesion 1	Spherical	4	30	50	60	50	0.4	1	0.04
	C_5	Lesion 2	Spherical	3	30	50	30	50	0.4	1	0.04

Figure 6-3(a) shows a schematic drawing of model I, where the single media dielectric object was placed at the center of a cube background. The target object has the dielectric properties of the human skin. The cube was made of lossless dielectric material ($\varepsilon_r = 36$) and it was placed at the window of the examination bed. The space between the window

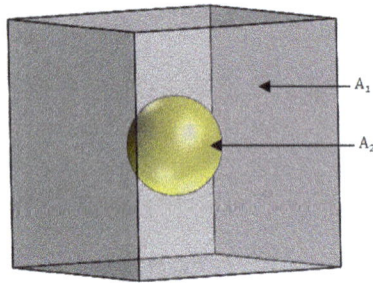

(a)

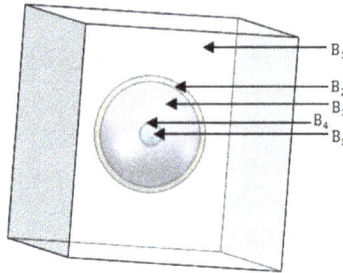

(b)

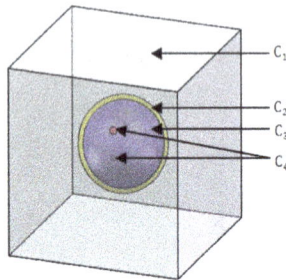

(c)

Figure 6-3 Models under test (a) Model I (b) Multimedia dielectric object II (c) Multimedia dielectric object III (A_1: background cube, A_2: skin, B_1: background cube, B_2: breast skin, B_3: breast fat, B_4: breast gland, B_5: breast lesion, C_1: background cube, C_2: breast skin, C_3: breast fat, C_4: breast lesion).

and the antenna array plane was filled with a lossless dielectric material ($\varepsilon_r = 36$). Figure 6-3(b) displays a schematic drawing of model II, where the multimedia dielectric object II is placed at the center of the cube. This multimedia object II was assumed as a breast that contains breast skin, fat, gland and one lesion. The scale values of the published dielectric properties of real breast tissues were applied to assume a small permittivity contrast between the object and the host medium as detailed above. Figure 6-3(c) shows a simulated model III, which was placed at the center of the cube. The object III was assumed as a breast that contains skin, fat, and two lesions. The distance between the two lesions was 1.27λ.

6.4   Simulation results

During simulation, one port of a microwave generator excites electromagnetic waves to the single transmitting antenna at a single frequency of 12.6 GHz ($\lambda = 23.8$ mm). The backscattered electric field from the target object was recorded at each receiver element on the array plane, which was connected to the second port of the microwave generator via a multi-position switch. The simulated backscattered field from the object then was applied to mapping the energy density of the object to produce a 2D image.

Figure 6-4(a) shows the original image of Model I. The cube image region (150 mm × 150 mm × 150 mm) containing the target object (Skin) and the background medium (lossless material close to skin) is uniformly subdivided into 60 × 60 × 60 elementary square cells. The modulus-part, real-part and imaginary-part of reconstructed images of model I are presented in Figures 6-4(b), (c), and (d). The simulation time was approximately 3.5 minutes for Model I.

Figure 6-5 shows the original image and 3D reconstructed images of model II. Model II contains a breast that is made of skin (5 mm thinness), fat, gland (10 mm in diameter), and one lesion (4 mm in diameter), where the breast model was located on the examination bed at $z = 0$ mm and the antenna array plane was placed at $z = -460$ mm and moved to $z = -440$ mm in 20 steps during screening. The cube image region (100 mm × 100 mm × 100 mm) containing the target object (breast) and the background medium (lossless material close to fat tissue) is uniformly subdivided into 80 × 80 × 80 elementary square cells. The total simulation time for Model II was approximately 10 minutes.

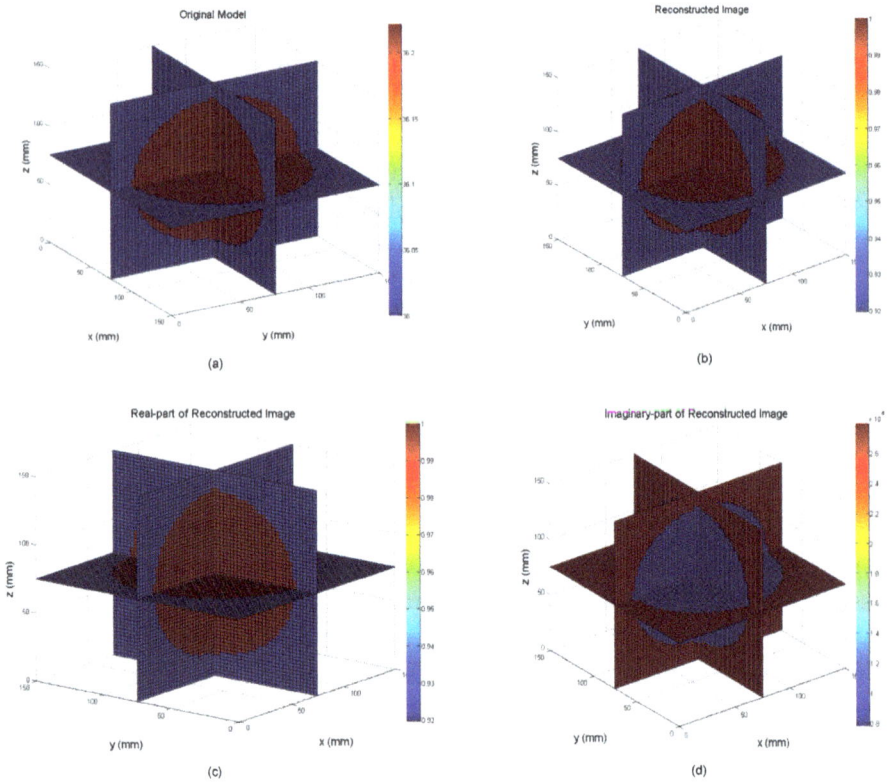

Figure 6-4 (a) Original image of object I (modulus-part) (b) 3D reconstructed image of object I (modulus-part) (c) reconstructed amplitude image (d) reconstructed phase image.

Figure 6-6(a) illustrates the original 3D image of the model III containing a breast and background cube (lossless material close to fat tissue). The breast contains skin (5 mm thinness), fat, and two lesions (3 mm and 4 mm in diameter, respectively). The image region (100 mm × 100 mm × 100 mm) is uniformly subdivided into 85 × 85 × 85 elementary square cells. Reconstructed images of model III are presented in Figure 6-6(b), (c) and (d). The total simulation time for model III was approximately 14.5 minutes.

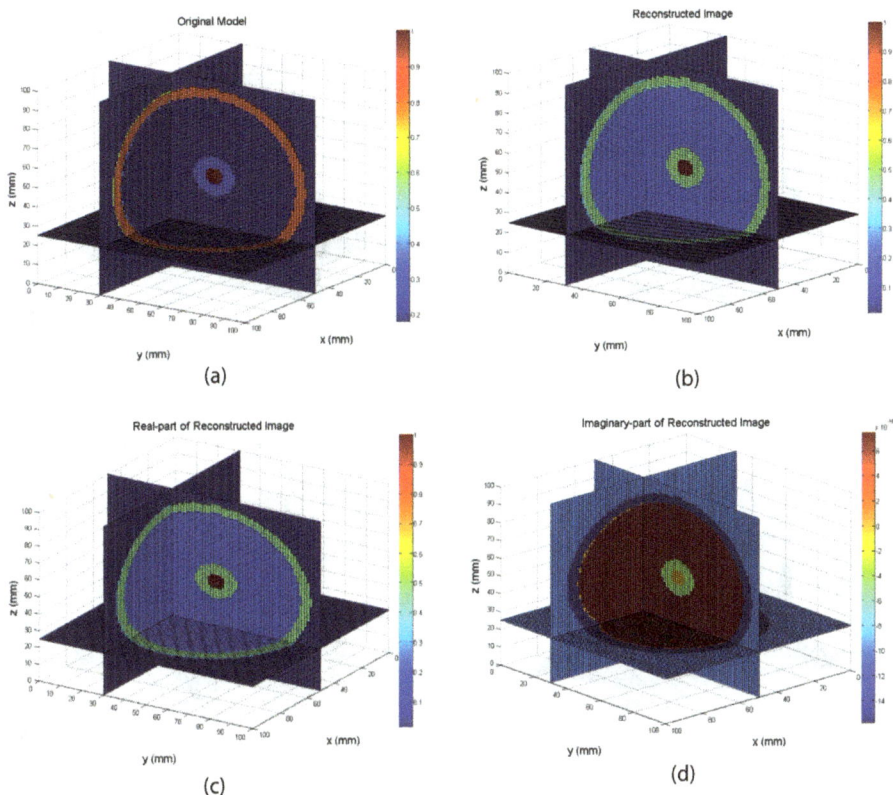

Figure 6-5 (a) Original image of object II (modulus value) (b) 3D reconstructed image of object II (modulus-part) (c) reconstructed amplitude image (d) reconstructed phase image.

Results demonstrated that all dielectric objects are successfully imaged and structures of objects are clearly identified. Small inclusions (lesion) within a multimedia dielectric object (breast) also fully imaged using the 3D HMI technique. In original images, color bars plot the dielectric properties (modulus value) of objects. In reconstructed images, color bars plot signal energy on a linear scale, normalized to the maximum in the 3D image space and values below 0.1 are rendered as blue.

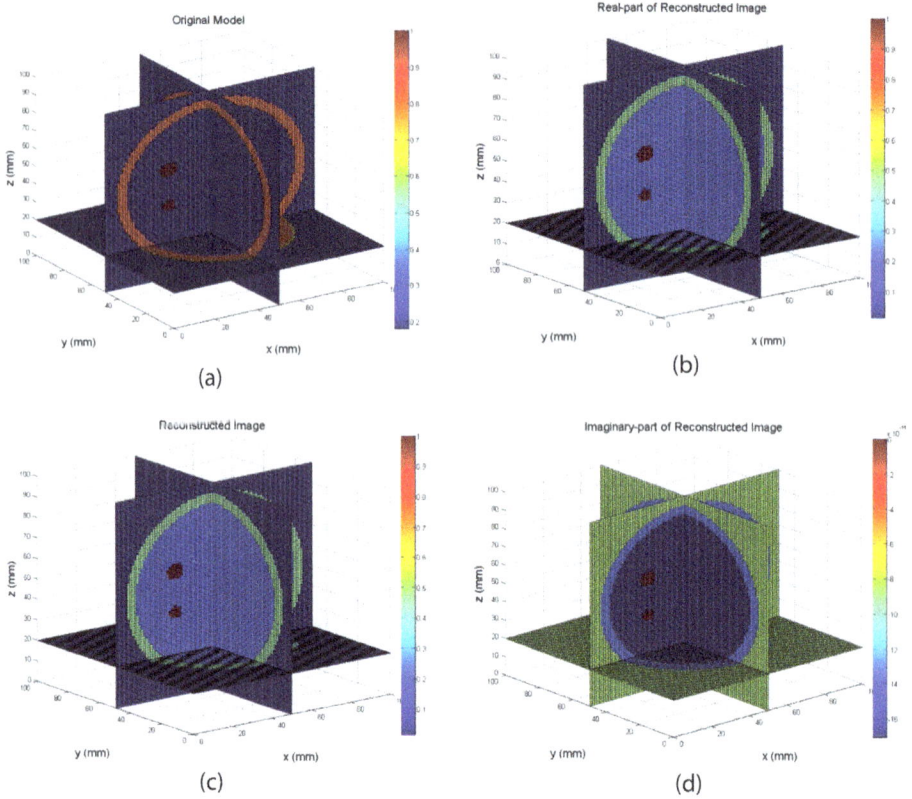

Figure 6-6 (a) Original image of object III (modulus-part) (b) 3D reconstructed image of object III (modulus-part) (c) reconstructed amplitude image (d) reconstructed phase image.

6.5 Closure

This chapter presented an application of the proposed technique. The contrast between breast lesion, fat tissue, gland and skin is very close to the real breast. The major limitation of the developed 2D imaging method is that only one object can be imaged if more than one object located at the same X and Y coordinates but at different Z-planes. Numerical results presented in this work demonstrate that multiple small inclusions (lesions) located at different locations within the object could be fully detected, which proves that the 3D imaging algorithm has an ability to solve the limitation of the 2D imaging technique.

7. Potential Application II-Brain stroke detection

This chapter presents the feasibility and potential performance characteristics of the proposed HMI technique for medical imaging applications, with a particular focus on head imaging and brain stroke detection. A computer simulation model was developed using MATLAB to validate the proposed theory.

7.1 Introduction

Brain stroke is the third leading cause of death after heart disease and cancer (Go et al., 2013). Brain stroke is the rapid loss of brain functions due to a disturbance in the blood supply. Ischemic strokes account for approximately 87% of all strokes. The risk factors for stroke include old age, hypertension, transient ischemic attack, diabetes, high cholesterol, cigarette smoking and atrial fibrillation (Mohammed et al., 2012). Several most commonly available medical imaging tools for stroke detection, they are Computed Tomography (CT), Magnetic resonant Imaging scanning (MRI), Positron Emission Tomography (PET) and ultrasound (Muir et al., 2006). But none of these tools is suitable for continuous monitoring of a stroke's evolution due to the high cost, time consuming imaging operations and the imaging equipment is not portable. CT imaging uses ionizing radiation that is harmful to the patient. Therefore, it is necessary to investigate new technologies that can improve the overall effectiveness of the diagnosis by using the existing medical imaging tools (Scapaticci et al., 2012).

7.2 Theory

Figure 7-1 shows the geometry of a 2D HMI. If two points $P(x,z)$ and $P'(x',z')$ are assumed in the head, then the backscattered electric field, E_{scat}, from the head at receiver, A_i, can be found by applying the 2D method of moments (MoM) (Harrington, 1993):

$$E_{scat}(r') = \frac{-jk_b^2}{4} \iint_A (\varepsilon(r) - \varepsilon_b) E_T(r) H_0^2(k_b R) dA \qquad (7\text{-}1)$$

Where
$E_{scat}(r')$ = scattered electric field at position, r
$j = \sqrt{-1}$
k_b = propagation constant in background medium
ε_b = complex relative permittivity of background medium

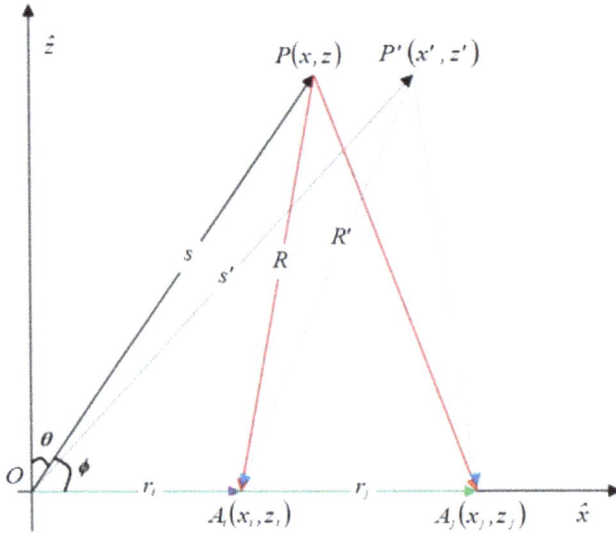

Figure 7-1 Geometry of HMI measurement by a pair of antennas.

$\varepsilon(r)$ = complex relative permittivity of head at position, r

$R = |r' - r|$ = distance between source point and field point

$E_T(r)$ = total electric field at position, r

$H_0^2(k_b R)$ = zero-order Hankel function of the second type with argument $k_b R$

A = area of head

d_A = differential area element

The total electric field of head is the sum of the scattered filed and the incident field:

$$E_T(r') = E_{scat}(r') + E_{inc}(r') \tag{7-2}$$

If assuming the field point at position, r', be a point inside the head, Equation (7-3) can be rewritten as:

$$E_{inc}(r') = E_T(r') - \frac{jk_b^2}{4}\iint_A (\varepsilon(r) - \varepsilon_b)E_T(r)H_0^2(k_b R)dA \tag{7-3}$$

The total field can be solved by using the Method of Moments (MoM) method to convert an integral equation into a set of linear simulation equations. Using the approach adopted by Richmond, the head area has been divided into small area element, ΔS, and the field and the permittivity is assumed constant with each ΔS. The integral in Equation (7-3) then becomes a sum over all the elemental areas. Equation (7-2) then becomes a matrix equation as follows:

$$[E_{inc}] = [[I] + [M]][E_T] = [Q][E_T] \tag{7-4}$$

Where $[Q] = [I] + [M]$
$[I]$ = Identity matrix $(N \times N)$
$[M]$ = Square matrix $(N \times N)$ with elements.

M_{mn} can be defined as follows (m = row index, n = column index). For the diagonal elements of $[M]$, that is, $m = n$

$$M_{mn} - (\varepsilon_n - \varepsilon_b)(1 + \frac{j\pi}{2}k_b H_1^2(k_b a) \tag{7-5}$$

For the off-diagonal elements of $[M]$, that is $m \neq n$

$$M_{mn} = \frac{jk_b^2}{4}\Delta S(\varepsilon_n - \varepsilon_b)H_0^2(k_b R_{mn}) \tag{7-6}$$

Where $\Delta S = \pi a^2$
$R_{mn} = |r_m - r_n|$
$H_1^2(k_b R)$ = First-order Hankel function of the second type with argument $k_b R$

The total field of equation (7-2) can be written as:

$$[E_T] = [Q]^{-1}[E_{inc}] \tag{7-7}$$

Submitting Equation (7-7) in (3-1):

$$G(r_i, r_j) = \left(\frac{-jk_b^2}{4}\right)^2 \iint_A \iint_{A'} |\varepsilon(r) - \varepsilon_b|^2 \tag{7-8}$$

$$E_T(r') \cdot E_T^*(r)H_0^2(k_b R)H_0^2(k_b R')dAdA'$$

Where $H_0^2(k_b R) \approx \sqrt{\dfrac{2}{\pi k_b R}} e^{-jk_b R} e^{j\pi/4}$

$H_0^2(k_b R') \approx \sqrt{\dfrac{2}{\pi k_b R'}} e^{-jk_b R'} e^{j\pi/4}$

If the distance from a point, P, to the receiving antenna, A_j, is sufficiently large to the size of antenna array plane, that is, $R \gg r_i$, then:

$$R = |R| \approx s - \frac{r_i \cdot s}{s} = s - r_i \cdot \hat{s} \qquad (7\text{-}9)$$

Similarly

$$R' = s' - r_j \cdot \hat{s'} \qquad (7\text{-}10)$$

Submitting (7-9) and (7-10) in (7-8), then

$$G(r_i, r_j) = \left(\frac{-jk_b^2}{4} \right) \iint_A |\varepsilon(r) - \varepsilon_b|^2 E_T(s) \cdot E_T^*(s) \frac{2 je^{-jk_b(r_i - r_j)\cdot \hat{s}}}{\pi k_b s} dA \quad (7\text{-}11)$$

$$= \left(\frac{jk_b}{2} \right)^3 \frac{1}{\pi} \iint_A |\varepsilon(r) - \varepsilon_b|^2 E_T(s) \cdot E_T^*(s) \frac{e^{-jk_b D \cdot \hat{s}}}{s} dA$$

Define the head intensity distribution as:

$$I(s) = \left(\frac{jk_b}{2} \right)^3 \frac{1}{\pi} |\varepsilon(r) - \varepsilon_b|^2 E_T(s) \cdot E_T^*(s) \qquad (7\text{-}12)$$

And defined the baseline vector, D_{ij}, of antenna, A_i, and antenna, A_j, as:

$$D_{ij} = \frac{r_j - r_i}{\lambda_b} \qquad (7\text{-}13)$$

Submitting Equation (7-12) and Equation (7-13) in Equation (7-11) and applying of spherical polar coordinate system, Equation (7-11) changes to the bellow (see Figure 7-1):

$$G(D_{ij}) = \int_l \int_m I(s) \frac{e^{-j2\pi D_{ij}\cdot \hat{s}}}{n} \, dl dm \qquad (7\text{-}14)$$

Where $l = \cos\phi$, $m = 0$, $n = \cos\theta = \sqrt{1-l^2}$, $\hat{s} = \cos\phi \hat{x} + \cos\theta \hat{z}$
The visibility function can be rewritten as:

$$G(u_{ij}) = \int_l \frac{I(s)}{\sqrt{1-l^2}} e^{-j2\pi \Phi_{ij}} \, dl \qquad (7\text{-}15)$$

Where $\Phi_{ij} = D \cdot \hat{s} = u_{ij}l$
$$u_{ij} = \frac{x_j - x_i}{\lambda_b}$$
λ_b = wavelength in background medium

Now define a line integral along the radial coordinate, s, so that:

$$\tilde{I}(l, m = 0) = \int_s \frac{I(s,l)}{\sqrt{1-l^2}} \, ds \qquad (7\text{-}16)$$

The complex visibility function becomes:

$$G(u_{ij}) = \int_l \tilde{I}(l) e^{-j2\pi u_{ij}l} \, dl \qquad (7\text{-}17)$$

Equation (7-17) is the 1D Fourier transform of the head intensity function, $\tilde{I}(l)$. The head intensity distribution function can be obtained by using an inverse Fourier transform:

$$\tilde{I}(l) = \int_u G(u_{ij}) e^{-j2\pi u_{ij}l} \, du \qquad (7\text{-}18)$$

The antenna array plane was designed and can be moved from H_1 to H_n in M steps during data collection, where H is the distance between the antenna array plane and the head. Then the tumor at the head z location, z_n, within the same head model was defined as:

$$z_n = s_n \cos\theta_n \qquad (7\text{-}19)$$

Where θ_n is the receiving angle of the same receiver on the receiving antenna array plane to the detected object at the position, s_n, with the receiving antenna array plane to the head at the distance, H_n. Thus, ds, in Equation (7-16) became:

$$ds = \frac{dz}{\cos\theta_n} = \frac{dz}{\sqrt{1-l^2}} \tag{7-20}$$

The backscattered electric field from the head at each height is collected, the 2D integral of the head intensity function through a selected height, $H = H_n$, can be obtained as:

$$I(H = z_n, l) = \frac{d\tilde{I}(l) \cdot (1-l^2)}{dz} \tag{7-21}$$

The head intensity integral difference at two different heights is calculated as:

$$I(H = z_n, l) - I(H = z_{n-1}, l) = \frac{\tilde{I}_{z_n} - \tilde{I}_{z_{n-1}}}{z_n - z_{n-1}} \tag{7-22}$$

A 2D reconstructed head image can be achieved by summing the integral difference (7-22) when the receiver array plane placed at difference heights:

$$\tilde{I}(H, l) = \sum_{z_1}^{z_n} \frac{\tilde{I}_{z_n} - \tilde{I}_{z_{n-1}}}{z_n - z_{n-1}} \tag{7-23}$$

7.2.1 Simulation setup

The 2D HMI technique for brain stroke detection is designed for operating at a single frequency of 2.5 GHz. Figure 7-2 illustrates the HMI system for a 2D head model. The system contains an array of 16 small antennas, one is the transmitter and others are receivers which are located around the head model in far-filed distance. The space between the head model and antenna array was filled with air.

Figure 7-3 shows a 2D ellipse-shaped head model that has a major radius of 100 mm and a minor radius of 85 mm. The simulated 2D head model contains skin, fat, skull, cerebral spin fluid (CSF), grey matter, white matter and an ischemic stroke area. Color bar plots the dielectric properties of the head. The head model was surrounded with air as well as the space between the head model and antenna array. The dielectric properties of the head model are summarized in Table 7-1 (Wang et al., 2013a).

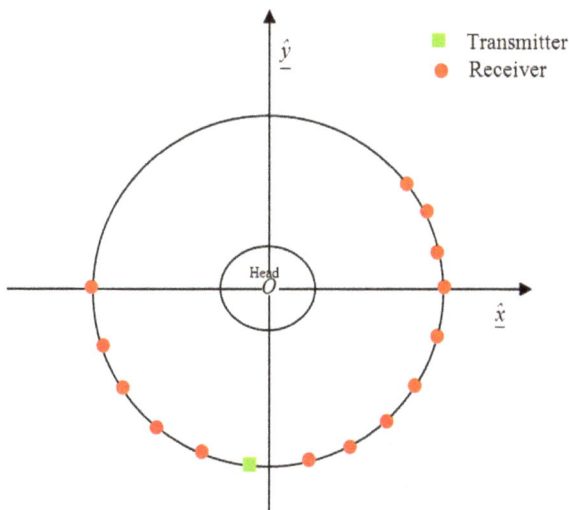

Figure 7-2 Schematic HMI system for 2D head model.

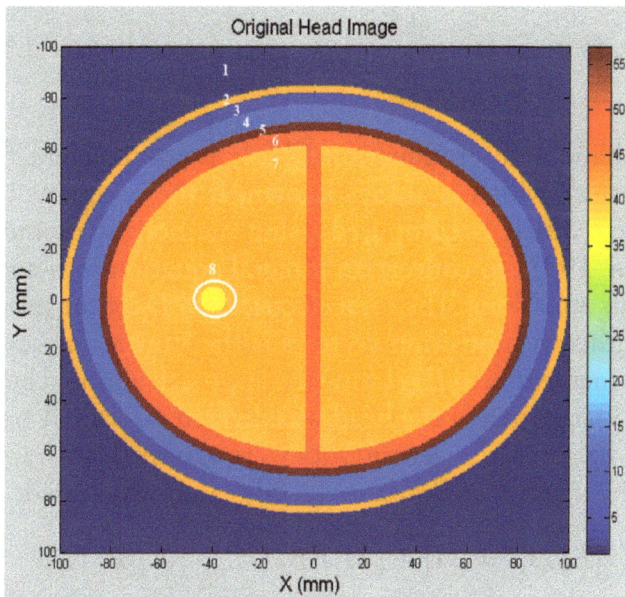

Figure 7-3 Simulated 2D head model inside of the HMI (1: air, 2: skin, 3: fat, 4: skull, 5: CSF, 6: grey matter, 7: white matter, 8: ischemic stroke).

Table 7-1 Dielectric properties of head at 2.5 GHz (Wang et al., 2013a).

No	Region	Thickness (mm)	Dielectric properties
1	Air		1 [38]
2	Skin	3	41-11j
3	Fat	5	5-4j
4	Skull	7	13-2j
5	CSF	3	57-26j
6	Grey matter	6	50-18j
7	White matter		40-15j
8	Ischemic stroke	5	36-13j

A wire antenna was simulated as the transmitter and receiver. The incident field of such antenna can be given by:

$$E_{inc}(s) = E_T(s) + \frac{jk_b^2}{4} \int_A (\varepsilon(s) - \varepsilon_b) E_T(s) H_0^2(k_b R) dA \qquad (7\text{-}24)$$

The left-hand side of Equation (7-24) is the incident field within the head model, which is always known. It then remains to solve the total field E_T which is computed using method of moment (MoM) (Harrington, 1993) to convert an integral equation into a set of linear simultaneous equations. The total electric field E_T of the head at a point inside the head with position vector s is the sum of the scattered filed E_{scat} and the incident field E_{inc}. Using the approach adopted by Richmond (Silver, 1949), the area of the head was divided into small area elements ΔS and the field and the permittivity were assumed constant with each ΔS. Then the integral in Equation (7-24) can be expressed:

$$[E_{inc}(s)] = [[I] + [M]][E_T(s)] = [Q][E_T(s)] \qquad (7\text{-}25)$$

Where $[Q] = [I] + [M]$, $[I]$ = Identity matrix $(N \times N)$, $[M]$ = Square matrix $(N \times N)$ with elements M_{mn} defined as follows (mm = row index, nn = column index).

The element of [M] is expressed as:

$$M_{mn} = \begin{cases} (\varepsilon_n(s) - \varepsilon_b)\left(1 + j\dfrac{\pi}{2}k_b H_1^2(k_b a)\right), \text{ for } m = n \\[4mm] \dfrac{jk_b^2}{4}\Delta S(\varepsilon_n(s) - \varepsilon_b)H_0^2(k_b R_{mn}), \text{ for } m \neq n \end{cases} \tag{7-26}$$

Where $a = \sqrt{\Delta S/\pi}$, and $H_1^2(k_b a)$ is the first-order Hankel function of the second type with argument $k_b a$, $\Delta S = \pi a$, and $R_{mn} = |r_m - r_n|$.

The total field can be found by matrix inversion of (7-26):

$$[E_T(s)] = [Q]^{-1}[E_{inc}(s)] \tag{7-27}$$

The backscattered electric field E_{scat} from the head at any receiver can be found using the MoM approach:

$$E_{scat}(r_i) = \left(-\dfrac{jk_b^2}{4}\right)\int_A |\varepsilon(s) - \varepsilon_b|E_T(s)H_0^2(k_b R)dA \tag{7-29}$$

Where $H_0^2(k_b R) \approx \sqrt{2/\pi k_b R}e^{-jk_b R}e^{j\pi/4}$, R is the position vector from a point in the head to the receiving antenna, A is head area and dA is differential area element.

An array of 16 wire antennas including one transmitter and 15 receivers (Figure 7-4) was placed around the head model in far-field (400 mm) distance.

A computer model was developed using MATLAB by combining Equation (7-28) and Equation (3-1) to simulate the complex visibility function. The head intensity distribution can be obtained by Equation (7-18) and then a 2D head image can be formed by Equation (7-22).

7.2.2 Simulation results

Figure 7-5 clearly shows the simulated ischemic stroke within the reconstructed 2D head image. The stroke is located at (X = −40 mm, Y = 0 mm). Color bar plots signal energy on a linear scale, normalized to the maximum in the 2D head area.

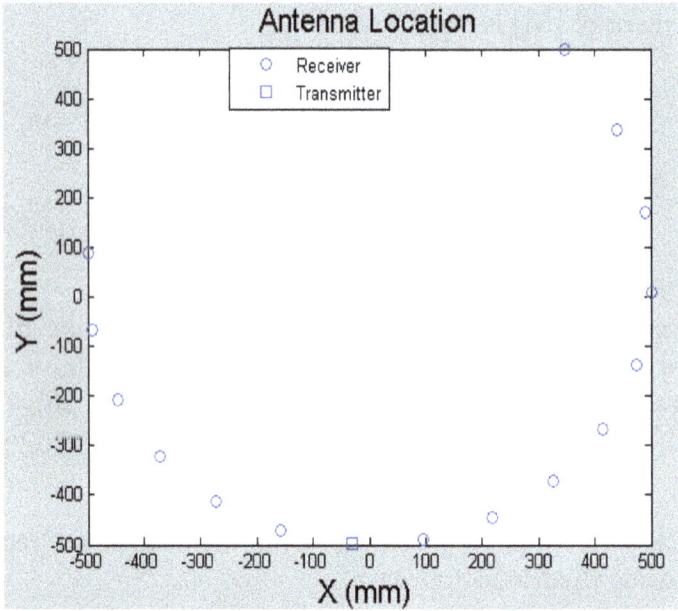

Figure 7-4   Schematic of antenna array configuration.

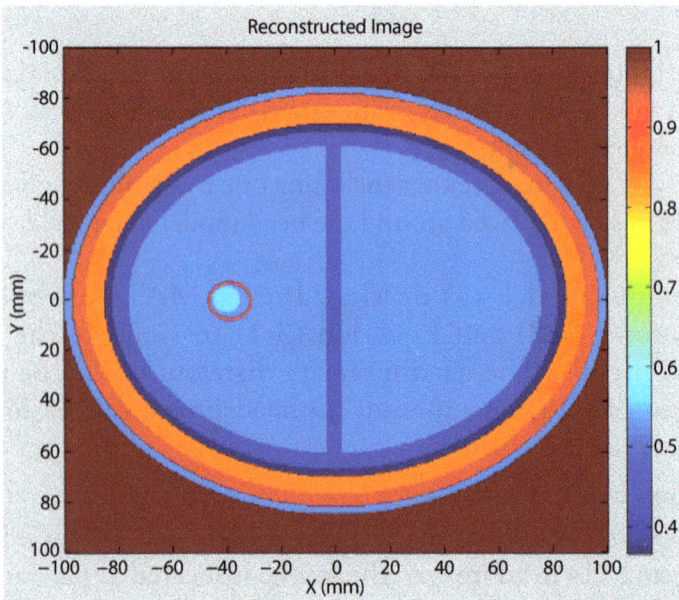

Figure 7-5   Reconstructed 2D head image of the simulated 2D head model.

7.3 Closure

An application of HMI technique for brain imaging and stroke detection was presented in this chapter. The 2D computational model was developed to demonstrate the proposed imaging technique. Simulation result showed that small stroke area (5 mm in diameter) inside of a high dielectric contrast shield, comprising the skull and cerebral spinal fluid could be detected. This technique has potential benefits in terms of significant improvement of imaging results, simplicity, safety and comfort compared to other screening modalities, such as X-ray.

8. Conclusions and future trends

8.1 Conclusions

This project investigated a new microwave imaging approach for detecting and imaging of dielectric objects, which may have potential applications in medical field in the future.

New 2D and 3D HMI image reconstruction algorithms that allows for the detection and localization of dielectric object responses were developed and demonstrated on a simplified dielectric model using MATLAB simulation environments. Simulation results demonstrated that as small as 2 mm in diameter anywhere within the 3D dielectric objects could be successfully detected. Simplified 2D and 3D HMI experimental systems were conducted to evaluate the theory. Experimental results showed that the 2D and 3D HMI techniques have capabilities for small inclusions (2.5 mm in diameter) detection within a dielectric object.

A flanged ORWA was designed for the experimental setups, which operated at 12.12 GHz for a return loss below -60 dB. The best performance of an array of 16 antennas was achieved at 12.6 GHz. The antenna was designed to radiate directly into air without a matching solution medium that has similar dielectric properties to breast tissue. Additionally, several antenna array configurations were investigated to produce a high-resolution image using the minimum number of antennas. Both simulation and experimental results showed that the proposed spiral and random antenna array configurations have the ability to produce high-resolution images compared to the currently widely used regularly spaced array, which can reduce the implementation costs and scanning time.

Various computer breast models were developed to demonstrate that the HMI techniques have the potential to detect breast lesions. Born approximation was used to solve the total electric field in the numerical simulations. Simulation results demonstrated that a small lesion would be detected using the proposed approach. Moreover, numerical head model was developed to demonstrate that the proposed 2D HMI technique has the potential to detect brain strokes. Different from the breast model, the Method of Moments approach was applied to solve the total electric field in the simulations. Simulation result showed that a small ischemic stroke area (5 mm in diameter) inside of a high dielectric contrast shield, comprising the skull and cerebral spinal fluid could be detected using the HMI approach.

Although a simplified phantom and a simple waveguide antenna were considered in this first generation experimental system, both simulation and experimental results proved that the developed 2D and 3D HMI techniques have the potential application in medical imaging fields such as breast image, head image. The benefits of HMI techniques including significant improvement of imaging results, simplicity, safety and comfort compared to other screening modalities, such as X-ray mammography.

8.2 Future trends

The major limitation of the HMI experimental setups includes a longer operation time was required to generate a good quality 3D image due to manual operation and manual height adjustment of the antenna array plane in the data collection processing. The CPU time required to calculate a 3D image (data collected at 49 different heights) was approximately 2 minutes on an Intel Xeon E5620 2.4 GHz with 18 GB RAM. This limitation will be solved in the future by developing a complex practical system to collect and store data automatically, and the initial design of such system was reported in Chapter 5.

Compared to other microwave imaging systems, the most significant benefit of the proposed technique is that 3D images with reasonable resolution can be obtained using data acquired at just one frequency, which simplified the experimental setups. Another potential benefit of the methodology is that the liquid matching medium was not required in the measurement system. This allows for a lower cost and easier setup for the experimental system. Additionally, the antenna array provides the maximum combination of receiving antennas and enables the collection of out of plane transmission data. For a single transmitter and 15 receivers, the total number of independent measurement points using the HMI technique is 210, but it is only 15 points for the same number of antennas using the microwave imaging approach detailed in (Klemm et al., 2011). This will improve the image quality for a given number of antennas, whilst reducing the cost.

Implementing the 3D HMI technique on real biological tissues is planned in the near future. The potential applications of this technique are most likely breast cancer detection, and brain stroke detection. An important issue that will need to be addressed in the future is the extension of the analysis to 3D phantoms with a realistic shape and realistic tissue architecture. In the case of breast cancer detection using the 3D HMI technique, further areas of study including:

- Development of a realistic breast phantom that is close to real human tissue architecture
- Development of a complex practical system to reduce the data acquisition time
- Further experiments on multiple realistic breast phantoms to investigate the performance of breast cancer detection using HMI algorithms
- Design and build a compact patch antenna array suitable for a clinical trial system setup
- Validation of the 3D HMI technique through measurement studies on living tissues and mastectomy tissue
- Comparison between HMI images and other microwave images, as well as existing medical imaging tools such as X-ray mammography and MRI.

References

Andreas, F., Mats, G., and Sven, N. (2012). "Image reconstruction in microwave tomography using a dielectric Debye model." *IEEE Transactions on Biomedical Engineering*, 59(1), 156–166.

Andrew, W. (2012). "Increasing the sensitivity of magnetic resonance spectroscopy and imaging." *Analytical Chemistry*, 84(1), 9–16.

Assmus, A. (1995). "Early history of X-rays." *Lie and Non-Lie Symmetries of Nonlinear Diffusion Equations with*, 25.

Badgwell, B.D., Giordano, S.H., Duan, Z.Z., Fang, S., Bedrosian, I., and Kuerer, H.M. (2008). "Mammography before diagnosis among women age 80 years and older with breast cancer." *Journal of Clinical Oncology*, 26(15), 2482–2488.

Bech, M., Jensen, T.H., Bunk, O., Donath, T., David, C., and Weitkamp, T. (2010). "Advanced contrast modalities for X-ray radiology: Phase-contrast and dark-field imaging using a grating interferometer." *Zeitschrift Für Medizinische Physik*, 20(1), 7–16.

Bihan, D.L., Mangin, J.F., Poupon, C., Clark, C.A., Pappata, S., Molko, N. (2001). "Diffusion tensor imaging: Concepts and applications." *Journal of Magnetic Resonance Imaging*, 13(4), 534–546.

Bindu, G., and Mathew, K.T. (2007). "Characterization of benign and malignant breast tissues using 2-D microwave tomographic imaging." *Microwave & Optical Technology Letters*, 49(10), 2341–2345.

Board, A.D.A.M.E. (2011). Arm CT scan. A.D.A.M.

Bond, E.J., Li, X., Hagness, S.C., and Van Veen, B.D. (2003). "Microwave imaging via space-time beamforming for early detection of breast cancer." *IEEE Transactions on Antennas & Propagation*, 51(8), 1690–1705.

Born, M., and Wolf, E. (1980). *Principles of Optics*. Pergamon Press, Sixth Edition, Chapter 10.4.2, 510.

Broquetas, A., Romeu, J., Rius, J.M., Elias-Fuste, A.R., Cardama, A., and Jofre, L. (1991). "Cylindrical geometry: A further step in active microwave tomography." *IEEE Transactions on Microwave Theory & Techniques*, 39(5), 836–844.

Cercignani, M., and Horsfield, M.A. (2001). "The physical basis of diffusion-weighted MRI." *Journal of the Neurological Sciences*, 186(1), S11–S14.

Chan, V., and Perlas, A. (2011). *Basics of Ultrasound Imaging*. Springer New York.

Colin, G., Puyan, M., Amer, Z., Majid, O., Cameron, K., and Sima, N. et al. (2010). "A wideband microwave tomography system with a novel frequency selection procedure." *IEEE Transactions on Biomedical Engineering*, 57(4), 894–904.

Craddock, I.J., Preece, A., Leendertz, J., Klemm, M., Nilavalan, R., and Benjamin, R. (2006). "Development of a hemi-spherical wideband antenna array for breast cancer imaging." *2006 European Conference on Antennas and Propagation EUCAP*, 6–10.

David, G., and Bruce, M. (2007). "MRI evaluation of breast cancer." *New England Journal of Medicine*, 357(2), 191–193.

Davis, T.J., Gao, D., Gureyev, T.E., Stevenson, A.W., and Wilkins, S.W. (1995). "Phase-contrast imaging of weakly absorbing materials using hard X-rays." *Nature*, 373(6515), 595–598.

Deighton, A.M. (2013). "Differentiating between healthy and malignant lymph nodes at microwave frequencies." *Undergrad. Res. Alberta*, 3(1).

Demi, M. (2014). "The basics of ultrasound." *Comprehensive Biomedical Physics*, 57(9), 297–322.

Dorria Saleh, S., Rasha Mohamed, K., Sahar Mahmoud, M., Lamiaa Adel, S., and Rasha, W. (2013). "Breast imaging in the young: The role of magnetic resonance imaging in breast cancer screening, diagnosis and follow-up." *Journal of Thoracic Disease*, 5 suppl 1(2), S9–S18.

Eleuterio, R., and Conceicao, R.C. (2015). "Initial study for detection of multiple lymph nodes in the axillary region using Microwave Imaging." *9th European Conference on Antennas and Propagation (EuCAP)*.

Elmore, J.G., Barton, M.B., Moceri, V.M., Polk, S., Arena, P.J., and Fletcher, S.W. (1998). "Ten-year risk of false positive screening mammograms and clinical breast examinations." *The New England Journal of Medicine*, 43(5), 1089–1096.

Epstein, N.R., Meaney, P.M., and Paulsen, K.D. (2014). "3D parallel-detection microwave tomography for clinical breast imaging." *Review of Scientific Instruments*, 85(12), 124704-124704-12.

Fear, E.C., and Stuchly, M.A. (2000). "Microwave breast cancer detection." *IEEE MTT-S International Microwave Symposium*, 2, pp. 1037–1040.

Fear, E.C., Hagness, S.C., Meaney, P.M., and Okoniewski, M. (2002a). "Enhancing breast tumor detection with near-field imaging." *IEEE Microwave Magazine*, 3(1), 48–56.

Fear, E.C., Sill, J., and Stuchly, M.A. (2003). "Experimental feasibility study of confocal microwave imaging for breast tumor detection." *IEEE Transactions on Microwave Theory & Techniques*, 51(3), 887–892.

Fear, E.C., Xu, L., Hagness, S.C., and Stuchly, M.A. (2002b). "Confocal microwave imaging for breast cancer detection: Localization of tumors in three dimensions." *IEEE Transactions on Biomedical Engineering*, 49(8), 812–822.

Ferrara, K.W., Borden, M.A., and Zhang, H. (2009). "Lipid-shelled vehicles: Engineering for ultrasound molecular imaging and drug delivery." *Accounts of Chemical Research*, 42(7), 881–892.

Foster, K.R., and Schwan, H.P. (1989). "Dielectric properties of tissues and biological materials: A critical review." *Critical Reviews in Biomedical Engineering*, 17(17), 25–104.

Gabriel, C., Gabriel, S., and Corthout, E. (1996a). "The dielectric properties of biological tissues: I. literature survey." *Physics in Medicine & Biology*, 41(11), 2231–2249.

Gabriel, S., Gabriel, C., and Lau, R.W. (1996b). "The dielectric properties of biological tissues: III parametric models for the dielectric spectrum of tissues." *Physics in Medicine & Biology*, 41(11), 2271–2293.

Go, A.S., Mozaffarian, D., Roger, V.L., Benjamin, E.J., Berry, J.D., Borden, W.B., and Turner, M.B. (2013). "Heart disease and stroke statistics—2013 update a report from the American Heart Association." *Circulation*, 127, e6–e245.

Hagness, S.C., Taflove, A., and Bridges, J.E. (1998). "Two-dimensional FDTD analysis of a pulsed microwave confocal system for breast cancer detection: Fixed-focus and antenna-array sensors." *IEEE Transactions on Biomedical Engineering*, 47(5), 783–791.

Hagness, S.C., Taflove, A., and Bridges, J.E. (1999). "Three-dimensional FDTD analysis of an ultra-wide band antenna-array element for confocal microwave imaging of nonpalpable breast tumors." *Antennas and Propagation Society International Symposium*, 3, 1886–1889.

Haidekker, M.A., and Dougherty, G. (2011). *Medical Imaging in the Diagnosis of Osteoporosis and Estimation of the Individual Bone Fracture Risk.* Springer Berlin.

Haidekker, M.A. (2013a). *Magnetic Resonance Imaging. Medical Imaging Technology.* Springer New York.

Haidekker, M.A. (2013b). *Medical Imaging Technology.* Springer New York.

Halter, R.J., Zhou, T., Meaney, P.M., Hartov, A., Barth, R.J. Jr, Rosenkranz, K.M., Wells, W.A., Kogel, C.A., Borsic, A., Rizzo, E.J., and Paulsen, K.D. (2009). "The correlation of in vivo and ex vivo tissue dielectric properties to validate electromagnetic breast imaging: initial clinical experience." *Physiological Measurement*, 30(6), S121–S136.

Harrington, R.F. (1993). *Field Computation by Moment Methods.* Wiley-IEEE Press.

Heil, J., Czink, E., Schipp, A., Sohn, C., Junkermann, H., and Golatta, M. (2012). "Detected, yet not diagnosed—Breast cancer screening with MRI mammography in high-risk women." *Breast Care*, 7(3), 236–239.

Henriksson, T., Klemm, M., Gibbins, D., and Leendertz, J. (2011). "Clinical trials of a multistatic UWB radar for breast imaging." *2011 Loughborough Antennas and Propagation Conference (LAPC)*, pp. 1–4.

Hou, M.F., Chuang, H.Y., Ou, Y.F., Wang, C.Y., Huang, C.L., and Fan, H.M. (2002). "Comparison of breast mammography, sonography and physical examination for screening women at high risk of breast cancer in Taiwan." *Ultrasound in Medicine & Biology*, 28(4), 415–420.

Huynh, P.T., Jarolimek, A.M., and Daye, S. (1998). "The false-negative mammogram." *Radiographics*, 18(5), 1137–1154.

Ibrahim, W.M.A., and Algabroun, H.M. (2008). "The Family Tree of Breast Microwave Imaging Techniques." *4th Kuala Lumpur International Conference on Biomedical Engineering. Springer Berlin Heidelberg.*

Jackson, V.P., Hendrick, R.E., Feig, S.A., and Kopans, D.B. (1993). "Imaging of the radiographically dense breast." *Radiology*, 188(2), 297–301.

Jacobi, J.H., and Larsen, L.E. (1978). "Microwave interrogation of dielectric targets. Part II: By microwave time delay spectroscopy." *Medical Physics*, 5(6), 509–513.

Jacobs, M.A., Ibrahim, T.S., and Ouwerkerk, R. (2007). "MR imaging: Brief overview and emerging applications1." *Radiographics*, 27(4), 1213–1229.

John, S., Mark, H., Paul, C., and Mahta, M. (2012). "A preclinical system prototype for focused microwave thermal therapy of the breast." *IEEE Transactions on Biomedical Engineering*, 59(9), 2431–2438.

Joines, W.T., Zhang, Y., Li, C., and Jirtle, R.L. (1994). "The measured electrical properties of normal and malignant human tissues from 50 to 900 MHz." *Medical Physics*, 21(4), 547–550.

Kalender, W.A., and Quick, H.H. (2011). "Recent advances in medical physics." *European Radiology*, 21(3), 501–504.

Kamal, R.M., Razek, N.M.A., Hassan, M.A., and Shaalan, M.A. (2007). "Missed breast carcinoma; why and how to avoid?" *Journal of the Egyptian National Cancer Institute*, 19(3), 178–194.

Keen, J.D., and Keen, J.E. (2008). "How does age affect baseline screening mammography performance measures? A decision model." *BMC Medical Informatics & Decision Making*, 8(22), 40.

Kiessling, F., Fokong, S., Koczera, P., Lederle, W., and Lammers, T. (2012). "Ultrasound microbubbles for molecular diagnosis, therapy, and theranostics." *Journal of Nuclear Medicine*, 53(3), 345–348.

Klemm, M., Gibbins, D., Leendertz, J., and Horseman, T. (2011). "Development and testing of a 60-element UWB conformal array for breast cancer imaging." *Proceedings of the 5th European Conference on Antennas and Propagation (EUCAP)*, 3077–3079.

Klemm, M., Leendertz, J.A., Gibbins, D., Craddock, I.J., Preece, A., and Benjamin, R. (2010). "Microwave radar-based differential breast cancer imaging: Imaging in homogeneous breast phantoms and low contrast scenarios." *IEEE Transactions on Antennas & Propagation*, 58(7), 2337–2344.

Kurrant, D.J., Fear, E.C., and Westwick, D.T. (2008). "Tumor response estimation in radar-based microwave breast cancer detection." *IEEE Transactions on Biomedical Engineering*, 55(55), 2801–2811.

Larsen, L.E., and Jacobi, J.H. (1978). "Microwave interrogation of dielectric targets. Part I: By scattering parameters." *Medical Physics*, 5(6), 500–508.

Larsen, L.E., and Jacobi, J.H. (1986). *Medical Applications of Microwave Imaging*. IEEE Press.

Lazebnik, M., Okoniewski, M., Booske, J.H., and Hagness, S.C. (2007a)."Highly accurate Debye models for normal and malignant breast tissue dielectric properties at microwave frequencies." *IEEE Microwave & Wireless Components Letters*, 17(12), 822–824.

Lazebnik, M., Popovic, D., Mccartney, L., Watkins, C., Lindstrom, M., and Harter, J. (2007b). "A large-scale study of the ultrawideband microwave dielectric properties of normal, benign and malignant breast tissues obtained from cancer surgeries." *Physics in Medicine & Biology*, 52(20), 6093–6115.

Levanda, R., and Leshem, A. (2010)."Synthetic aperture radio telescopes." *IEEE Signal Processing Magazine*, 27(1), 14–29.

Li, X., and Hagness, S.C. (2001). "A confocal microwave imaging for breast cancer detection." *IEEE Microwave & Wireless Components Letters*, 11(3), 130–132.

Li, X., Davis, S.K., Hagness, S.C., Van, D.W.D.W., and Van Veen, B.D. (2004). "Microwave imaging via space-time beam forming: Experimental investigation of tumor detection in multilayer breast phantoms." *IEEE Transactions on Microwave Theory & Techniques*, 52(8), 1856–1865.

Magland, J.F., Wald, M.J., and Wehrli, F.W. (2009)."Spin-echo micro-MRI of trabecular bone using improved 3D fast large-angle spin-echo (flase)." *Magnetic Resonance in Medicine*, 61(61), 1114–1121.

Margarido, C., Arzola, C., MrinaliniBalki, and Carvalho, J.A. (2010). "No McCollough effect in a patient with cerebral achromatopsia but spared v1." *Journal of Vision*, 8(6), 489–489.

Meaney, P.M., Douglas, G., Golnabi, A.H., Tian, Z., Matthew, P., and Geimer, S.D. (2012a). "Clinical microwave tomographic imaging of the calcaneus: A first-in-human case study of two subjects." *IEEE Transactions on Biomedical Engineering*, 59(12), 3304–3313.

Meaney, P.M., Fanning, M.W., Raynolds, T., Fox, C.J., Fang, Q., and Kogel, C.A. (2007). "Initial clinical experience with microwave breast imaging in women with normal mammography." *Academic Radiology*, 14(2), 207–218.

Meaney, P.M., Zhou, T., Goodwin, D., Golnabi, A., Attardo, E.A., and Paulsen, K.D. (2012b). "Bone dielectric property variation as a function of mineralization at microwave frequencies." *International Journal of Biomedical Imaging*, 2012, 649612.

Mohammed, B.A.J., Abbosh, A.M., Ireland, D., and Bialkowski, M.E. (2012). "Compact wideband antenna for microwave imaging of brain." *Progress in Electromagnetics Research C*, 27, 27–39.

Muir, K.W., Buchan, A., von Kummer, R., Rother, J., and Baron, J.C. (2006). "Imaging of acute stroke." *The Lancet Neurology*, 5, 755–768.

Nikolova, N.K. (2011). "Microwave imaging for breast cancer." *IEEE Microwave Magazine*, 12(12), 78–94.

Ogawa, S., Lee, T.M., Kay, A.R., and Tank, D.W. (1990). "Brain magnetic resonance imaging with contrast dependent on blood oxygenation." *Proceedings of the National Academy of Sciences of the United States of America*, 87(24), 9868–9872.

O'Halloran, M., Conceicao, R.C., Byrne, D., Glavin, M., and Jones, E. (2009). "FDTD modeling of the breast: A review." *Progress in Electromagnetics Research B*, 18, 1–24.

O'Rourke, A.P., Mariya, L., Bertram, J.M., Converse, M.C., Hagness, S.C., and Webster, J.G. (2007). "Dielectric properties of human normal, malignant and cirrhotic liver tissue: In vivo and ex vivo measurements from 0.5 to 20 GHz using a precision open-ended coaxial probe." *Physics in Medicine and Biology*, 52(15), 4707–4719.

Pethig, R. (1984). "Dielectric properties of biological materials: Biophysical and medical applications." *IEEE Transactions on Electrical Insulation*, ei-19(5), 453–474.

Pfeiffer, F., Bech, M., Bunk, O., Kraft, P., Eikenberry, E.F., and Ch, B. et al. (2008). "Hard-x-ray dark-field imaging using a grating interferometer." *Nature Materials*, 7(2), 134–137.

Piccoli, C.W. (1997). "Contrast-enhanced breast MRI: Factors affecting sensitivity and specificity." *European Radiology*, 7(5), S281–S288.

Pichot, C., Jofre, L., Peronnet, G., and Bolomey, J.C. (1985). "Active microwave imaging of inhomogeneous bodies." *IEEE Transactions on Antennas & Propagation*, 33(4), 416–425.

Prinz, C., and Voigt, J.U. (2011). "Diagnostic accuracy of a hand-held ultrasound scanner in routine patients referred for echocardiography." *Journal of the American Society of Echocardiography*, 24(2), 111–116.

Radon, J. (1917). "Über die bestimmung von funktionen durch ihre in-te-gral-werte längs gewisser mannigfaltigkeiten." *Computed Tomography*, 69, 262–277.

Ron, E. (2003). "Cancer risks from medical radiation." *Health Physics*, 85(1), 47–59.

Rubæk, T. (2008). "Microwave imaging for breast-cancer screening." PhD Thesis.

Sadigh, G., Kelly, A.M., Fagerlin, A., and Carlos, R.C. (2011). "Patient preferences in breast cancer screening." *Academic Radiology*, (11), 1333–1336.

Said, T., and Varadan, V.V. (2009). "Variation of Cole-Cole model parameters with the complex permittivity of biological tissues," 2009. MTT '09. *IEEE International Microwave Symposium Digest MTT-S*, pp. 1445–1448.

Salvador, S.M., Fear, E.C., Okoniewski, M., and Matyas, J.R. (2010). "Exploring joint tissues with microwave imaging." *IEEE Transactions on Microwave Theory & Techniques*, 58(8), 2307–2313.

Scapaticci, R., Di Donato, L., Catapano, I., and Crocco, L. (2012). "A feasibility study on microwave imaging for brain stroke monitoring." *Progress in Electromagnetics Research B*, 40, 305–324.

Schepps, J.L., and Foster, K.R. (1980). "The uhf and microwave dielectric properties of normal and tumour tissues: Variation in dielectric properties with tissue water content." *Physics in Medicine & Biology*, 25(6), 1149–1159.

Semenov, S. (2009). "Microwave tomography: Review of the progress towards clinical applications." *Philosophical Transactions*, 367(1900), 3021–3042.

Semenov, S.Y., Svenson, R.H., Boulyshev, A.E., Souvorov, A.E., Borisov, V.Y., and Sizov, Y. (1996). "Microwave tomography: Two-dimensional system for biological imaging." *IEEE Transactions on Biomedical Engineering*, 43(9), 869–877.

Semenov, S.Y., Svenson, R.H., Bulyshev, A.E., Souvorov, A.E., Nazarov, A.G., and Sizov, Y.E. (2000). "Microwave spectroscopy of myocardial ischemia and infarction. 2. biophysical reconstruction." *Annals of Biomedical Engineering*, 28(1), 48–54.

Sha, L., Ward, E.R., and Stroy, B. (2002). "A review of dielectric properties of normal and malignant breast tissue." *SoutheastCon, 2002. Proceedings IEEE*, 457–462.

Silver, S. (1984). "Radiation from current distributions. Microwave Antenna Theory and Design." *IET Digital Library.*

Smart, C.R. (1997). "Limitations of the randomized trial for the early detection of cancer." *Cancer*, 79(9), 1740–1746.

Smith, D., Leach, M., and Kellner, A. (2004). "Indirect holographic imaging of antennas using an electronically synthesised 'slow-wave.'" *Antennas and Propagation Society International Symposium*, 1, 703–706.

Smith, D., Yurduseven, O., Livingstone, B., and Schejbal, V. (2014). "Microwave imaging using indirect holographic techniques." *IEEE Antennas & Propagation Magazine*, 56(1), 104–117.

Sunaga, T., Ikehira, H., Furukawa, S., Skinkai, H., Kobayashi, H., and Matsumoto, Y. (2002). "Measurement of the electrical properties of human skin and the variation among subjects with certain skin conditions." *Physics in Medicine & Biology*, 47(1), N11–N15(5).

Tilman, D., Franz, P., Oliver, B., Christian, G., Eckhard, H., and Stefan, P. (2010). "Toward clinical x-ray phase-contrast CT: Demonstration of enhanced soft-tissue contrast in human specimen." *Investigative Radiology*, 45(7), 445–52.

Wang, L., Simpkin, R., and Al-Jumaily, A.M. (2013a). "Holographic microwave imaging for medical applications." *Journal of Biomedical Science & Engineering*, 6(8), 823–833.

Wang, L., Al-Jumaily, A.M., and Simpkin, R. (2013b). "Holographic microwave imaging array for brain stroke detection." *Journal of Signal & Information Processing*, 4(3B), 96–101.

Wang, L., Simpkin, R., and Al-Jumaily, A.M. (2013c). "Open-ended waveguide antenna for microwave breast cancer detection." *2013 IEEE International Workshop on Electromagnetics (iWEM)*, 65–68.

Wang, L., Al-Jumaily, A.M., and Simpkin, R. (2014a). "Imaging of 3-D dielectric objects using far-field holographic microwave imaging technique." *Progress in Electromagnetics Research B*, 61, 135–147.

Wang, L., Simpkin, R., and Al-Jumaily, A.M. (2014b). "Three-dimensional far-field holographic microwave imaging: An experimental investigation of dielectric object." *Progress in Electromagnetics Research B*, 61, 169–184.

Wang, L., Al-Jumaily, A.M., and Simpkin, R. (2015). "Investigation of antenna array configurations using far-field holographic microwave imaging technique." *Progress in Electromagnetics Research M*, 42, 1–11.

Wehrli, F.W., Saha, P.K., Gomberg, B.R., Hee Kwon, S., Snyder, P.J., and Maria, B. (2002). "Role of magnetic resonance for assessing structure and function of trabecular bone." *Topics in Magnetic Resonance Imaging TMRI*, 13(5), 335–355.

Weitkamp, T. (2006). "Phase retrieval and differential phase-contrast imaging with low-brilliance X-ray sources." *Nature Physics*, 2(4), 258–261.

Author biography

Lulu Wang received her B.E. (honors) in Electronics and Computer Engineering from Manukau Institute of Technology, New Zealand, in 2008. Lulu obtained her M.E. (1st class honors) and PhD from Auckland University of Technology, New Zealand, in 2009 and 2013, respectively. After spending two years as a research follow at Institute of Biomedical Technologies, Auckland University of Technology, New Zealand, she moved to China. Lulu currently holds the post of Associate Professor at Hefei University of Technology, China. Lulu's current research focuses upon microwave sensing and imaging, MRI-informed functional imaging and continuous positive airway pressure therapy.

Lulu is a member of several professional societies, including American Society of Mechanical Engineers (ASME), Institute of Electrical and Electronics Engineers (IEEE), the American Association for the Advancement of Science (AAAS), Physiological Society of New Zealand (PSNZ) and Institution of Professional Engineers New Zealand (IPNZ). She currently serves as a Topic Organizer of ASME International Mechanical Engineering Congress and Exposition.

www.ingramcontent.com/pod-product-compliance
Lightning Source LLC
Chambersburg PA
CBHW050451190326
41458CB00005B/1238